前　言

《循证针灸临床实践指南》包括：带状疱疹、贝尔面瘫、抑郁症、中风后假性球麻痹、偏头痛、颈椎病、慢性便秘、腰痛、原发性痛经、坐骨神经痛、失眠、成人支气管哮喘、肩周炎、膝关节炎、急慢性胃炎、过敏性鼻炎、突发性耳聋、三叉神经痛、糖尿病周围神经病变、单纯性肥胖病等病症的循证针灸临床实践指南。

本部分为《循证针灸临床实践指南》的偏头痛部分。

本部分受国家中医药管理局指导与委托。

本部分由中国针灸学会提出。

本部分由中国针灸学会标准化工作委员会归口。

本部分起草单位：中国中医科学院针灸研究所。

本部分主要起草人：吴中朝、王京京、胡静、焦玥、周文娜、黄子明。

本部分专家组成员：刘保延、赵宏、武晓冬、房繄恭、赵吉平、刘志顺、吴泰相、杨金洪、梁繁荣、张维、刘炜宏、杨金生、文碧玲、余曙光、郭义、杨骏、赵京生、杨华元、储浩然、石现、王富春、王麟鹏、贾春生、余晓阳、高希言、常小荣、张洪涛、吕明庄、王玲玲、宣丽华、翟伟、岗卫娟、王昕、董国锋、王芳。

本部分首次发布于2011年，本次为第一次修订。

引　言

　　《循证针灸临床实践指南》是根据针灸临床优势，针对特定临床情况，参照古代文献、名医经验以及现代最佳临床研究证据，结合患者价值观和意愿，系统研制的帮助临床医生和患者做出恰当针灸处理的指导性意见。

　　《循证针灸临床实践指南》制定的总体思路是：在针灸实践与临床研究的基础上，遵循循证医学的理念与方法，紧紧围绕针灸临床的特色优势，综合专家经验、目前最佳证据以及患者价值观，将国际公认的证据质量评价与推荐方案分级的规范与古代、前人、名老针灸专家临床证据相结合，并将临床研究证据与大范围专家共识相结合，旨在制定出能保障针灸临床疗效和安全性，并具有科学性与实用性的可有效指导针灸临床实践的指导性意见。

　　在《循证针灸临床实践指南》的制定过程中，各专家组共同参与，还完成了国家标准《针灸临床实践指南制定与评估规范》（以下简称《规范》）的送审稿。《规范》参照了国际上临床实践指南制定的要求和经验，根据中国国情以及针灸的发展状况，对《循证针灸临床实践指南》制定的组织、人员、过程、采用证据质量评价、推荐方案等级划分、专家共识形成方式、制定与更新的内容和时间等都进行了规范。这些规范性要求在《指南》制定中都得到了充分考量与完善。《规范》与《循证针灸临床实践指南》相辅相成，《规范》是《循证针灸临床实践指南》制定的指导，《循证针灸临床实践指南》又是《规范》适用性的验证实例。

　　《循证针灸临床实践指南》推荐等级主要采用世界卫生组织（WHO）等推荐的 GRADE（Grading of Recommendations Assessment，Development and Evaluation）系统，即推荐分级的评价、制定与评估的系统，其中推荐等级分为强推荐与弱推荐两级。强推荐的方案是估计变化可能性较小，个性化程度低的方案，而弱推荐方案则是估计变化可能性较大，个性化程度高，患者价值观差异大的方案。对于古代文献和名医经验的证据质量评价，目前课题组还在进一步研制中，本《指南》仅将古代文献和名医经验作为证据之一附列在现代证据后面，供《循证针灸临床实践指南》使用者参考。

　　2008 年，在 WHO 西太区的项目资助下，由中国中医科学院牵头、中国针灸学会标准化工作委员会组织完成了针灸治疗带状疱疹、贝尔面瘫、抑郁症、中风后假性球麻痹和偏头痛 5 种病症的指南研制工作。在这 5 种病症的指南研制过程中，课题组初步提出了《循证针灸临床实践指南》的研究方法和建议，建立了《循证针灸临床实践指南》的体例、研究模式与技术路线。2010 年 12 月，《临床病症中医临床实践指南·针灸分册》由中国中医药出版社正式出版发行。

　　2009 年至 2013 年，在国家中医药管理局立项支持下，中国针灸学会标准化工作委员会又先后分3 批启动了 15 种病症的指南研制工作。为了保证《循证针灸临床实践指南》高质量地完成，在总课题组的组织下，由四川大学华西医院吴泰相教授在京举办两次 GRADE 方法学培训会议，全国 11 家临床及科研单位的 100 多位学员接受了培训。随后，总课题组又组织了 15 个疾病临床指南制定课题组和 1 个方法学课题组中的 17 位研究人员，赴华西医院循证医学中心接受了为期 3 个月的 Meta 分析和 GRADE 方法学专题培训，受训研究人员系统学习并掌握了 GRADE 系统证据质量评价和推荐意见形成的方法。

　　本次出版的《循证针灸临床实践指南》共有 20 个部分，包括对 2010 年版 5 部分指南的修订再版和 2013 年完成的 15 部分指南的首次出版。《循证针灸临床实践指南》的适用对象为从事针灸临床与科研的专业人员。

《循证针灸临床实践指南》的证据质量分级和推荐强度等级如下：

◇证据质量分级

证据质量高：A

证据质量中：B

证据质量低：C

证据质量极低：D

◇推荐强度等级

支持使用某项干预措施的强推荐：1

支持使用某项干预措施的弱推荐：2

《循证针灸临床实践指南》的编写，凝聚着全国针灸标准化科研人员和管理人员的辛勤汗水，是参与研制各方集体智慧的结晶，是辨证论治的个体化诊疗模式与循证医学有机结合的创造性探索。《循证针灸临床实践指南》在研制过程中，得到了兰州大学循证医学中心杨克虎教授、陈耀龙博士以及北京大学循证医学中心詹思延教授在方法学上的大力支持和帮助，在此深表感谢。同时，还要感谢国家中医药管理局政策法规与监督司领导的热心指导与大力支持；此外，还要感谢各位专家的通力合作；在《循证针灸临床实践指南》的出版过程中，中国中医药出版社表现出了很高的专业水平，在此一并致谢。

摘　　要

1　治疗原则

治疗原则：行气活血、疏通少阳为主。发作期通络止痛、辨经论治为主；缓解期疏通经络，配合辨证论治、综合各种针灸疗法。

取穴原则：发作期以少阳经穴、阿是穴为主，配合辨经取穴及耳穴。缓解期在发作期取穴基础上结合辨证配穴。

2　主要推荐意见

推荐意见	推荐级别
发作期针灸方案	
（1）放血治疗 　发作期偏头痛推荐首先使用局部刺络，耳轮或耳背上 1/3 有络脉或者全身症状明显者可同时配合耳郭刺血。缓解期肝阳上亢、瘀血型患者也可参照治疗	强推荐
（2）针刺（电针）治疗 　发作期偏头痛推荐以少阳经穴为主，配合经络辨证取穴，可用透穴针刺结合阿是穴电针治疗	强推荐
（3）火针治疗 　发作期偏头痛在针刺治疗基础上，可配合使用火针治疗	弱推荐
临床缓解期针灸方案	
综合针灸治疗 　缓解期偏头痛推荐以少阳经穴为主，兼顾经络、脏腑辨证取穴的毫针刺法，可同时配合头针、电针、温针灸、放血等治疗	强推荐

简　介

《循证针灸临床实践指南：偏头痛》（以下简称《指南》）简介如下：

1　本《指南》制定的目标

基于循证医学方法研究及专家意见共识，为临床医生提供治疗偏头痛高质量的针灸方案。

2　本《指南》制定的目的

促进国内偏头痛针灸治疗方案的规范化，为临床医生提供针灸治疗偏头痛的可靠性证据，以确保治疗的有效性及安全性。

3　本《指南》的适用人群

主要为执业中医师、执业助理中医师、非针灸专业的医务人员、患者，以及针灸科研人员。

本《指南》适用的目标环境包括国内各级医院针灸科门诊部或住院部，以及有针灸专业医师的基层、社区、医院科室和医院，各针灸相关的科研及评价机构。

4　本《指南》适用的疾病范围

本《指南》的目标疾病是偏头痛，由于先兆偏头痛和无先兆偏头痛在偏头痛中占绝大多数，且在相关针治文献中，绝大部分针对这两型，故《指南》仅针对这两型偏头痛进行针灸治疗方案推荐。其他类型偏头痛，或其他原发性和继发性头痛，也可以参考推荐方案辨证施治。

本《指南》主要适用于成人，适宜的介入时期可以在偏头痛发作期和缓解期。特殊人群（如儿童）偏头痛，也可以参考推荐方案辨证施治。

概　述

1　定义

1.1　西医

偏头痛是一种常见的神经血管性疾患，以反复发作的一侧或双侧搏动性头痛为特点，发作时多有自主神经症状，如恶心呕吐，面色苍白，心率及呼吸增快、胃肠道功能紊乱等。多于儿童期和青春期起病，中青年期达发病高峰。女性多见，常与月经周期有关。约60%的偏头痛患者有家族史。

1.2　中医

偏头痛属于中医学的"头风"范畴，以反复发作、或左或右、来去突然的剧烈头痛为主要表现，有时表现为周期性呕吐或腹痛。本病在中医古代文献中多被称为"偏头风""偏正头风""偏头痛""偏正头痛""头偏痛""偏头风痛""头半寒痛""脑风"。

2　发病率及人群分布情况

流行病学调查显示，偏头痛呈一种分布不均衡的高发状态：西方国家发病率较高，欧美国家为1500～2000/10万人，中国为732.1/10万人[1]；女性发病率高于男性，男女患者的比例国外为1∶2～3，中国为1∶4。白人的偏头痛发病率最高，非洲裔其次，亚洲裔最低[2]。偏头痛可发生于任何年龄，多在儿童期和青春期起病，首次发作在青春期附近有一高峰。中青年期（40岁左右）达发病高峰，以后逐渐下降。患病年龄，国外以25～45岁多见，中国以20～45岁多见[3]。2011年中国一项偏头痛流行病学研究表明：本病人群患病率为9.3%，男性为5.0%～6.9%，女性为11.5%～14.1%，全国年花费可达3317亿元人民币[4]。

临床特点

1 病史

偏头痛具有家族发病倾向，2/3 的病例都有家族遗传的因素[5]，虽然偏头痛很少是因为一种基因缺陷而导致的[6]，但可以认为某些个体的高度易感状态是促使该病发生的重要条件。比起无先兆偏头痛，这种遗传关系在有先兆偏头痛中表现得更为明显。母亲的遗传因素强于父亲。双亲患有偏头痛时，子女发病率为 75%；近亲有偏头痛时，发病率为 50%；远亲有偏头痛时，发病率为 20%。

偏头痛也具有显著的性别差异，在青春期之前，受到偏头痛影响的男童比女童要稍多，但在此之后，受到偏头痛影响的女性则比男性要多出两至三倍。通常在怀孕期间，偏头痛的影响会减弱[7,8]。

2 症状及体征

偏头痛通常是局部、反复发作和自限性的严重头痛，并伴有自主神经系统的相关症状[5]。有偏头痛史的人群中有 15%～30% 都有病发先兆[9]，并且有偏头痛病发先兆的人群，还经常出现无先兆即发病的情况。疼痛剧烈程度、头痛持续时间和发作频率则因人而异[5]。

偏头痛发作可分为前驱期、先兆期、头痛期和恢复期，但并非所有患者或所有发作均具有上述四期。同一患者可有不同类型的偏头痛发作[10]。

2.1 前驱期

前驱症状，即在头痛发作几小时前甚至几天前的症状，见于约 60% 的偏头痛患者[11]，这些症状可能包括各种情况，如激惹、情绪变化、疲倦、特别希望吃到某种食物、反复哈欠、活动少、肌肉僵硬（特别是颈部肌肉）、便秘或腹泻、对某种气味或噪音敏感等[12]。无论有无先兆偏头痛均有可能出现这些症状[13]，但常被患者忽略。

2.2 先兆期

"先兆"指头痛发作之前出现的可逆的局灶性脑功能异常症状，可为视觉性、感觉性或语言性。多数患者先兆期没有明显症状，只有先兆偏头痛等少数类型有先兆症状。先兆症状可持续数分钟到 1 小时，复杂性偏头痛病例的先兆期可持续较长时间。有些病人只有先兆症状而无头痛发作，即为偏头痛等位症。先兆症状主要包括：

视觉先兆：最为常见，典型的表现为闪光性暗点，如注视点附近出现"之"字形闪光，并逐渐向周边扩展，随后出现"锯齿形"暗点。有些患者可能仅有暗点，而无闪光。其他先兆还有畏光、视幻觉、水波纹、城垛形、视野缺损、视物变形、物体颜色改变、同向性偏盲等，可持续 20～30 分钟。

感觉先兆：表现为以面部和上肢为主的针刺感、麻木感或蚁行感。

先兆期其他症状较少出现，包括言语障碍、眩晕，以及不太常见的肢体协调困难。

2.3 头痛期

约 60% 的头痛发作以单侧为主，可左右交替发生，约 40% 为双侧头痛。头痛多位于颞部，也可位于前额、枕部或枕下部。偏头痛的头痛有一定的特征，程度多为中至重度，性质多样但以搏动性最具特点。头痛常影响患者的生活和工作，行走、登楼、咳嗽或打喷嚏等简单活动均可加重头痛，故患者多喜卧床休息。

偏头痛发作时，常伴有食欲下降，约 2/3 的患者伴有恶心，重者呕吐。尚可伴有感知觉增强，表现为对光线、声音和气味敏感，喜欢黑暗、安静的环境。其他较为少见的表现有头晕、直立性低血压、易怒、言语表达困难、记忆力下降、注意力不集中等。部分患者在发作期会出现由正常的非致痛性刺激所产生的疼痛。

成年人的头痛时间通常持续 4～72 小时[14]，但儿童的头痛持续时间则通常少于 1 小时[15]。头痛发作频率因人而异，有的人可能一生只发生几次，有的人则可能一周发作好几次，而平均水平为每个月一次[16]。

2.4 恢复期

头痛在发作后可自行缓解，但患者还可出现一些后遗症状：如疲劳、倦怠、易怒、不安、食欲差、注意力不集中、头皮触痛、欣快、抑郁或其他不适，影响可能会持续几天。

诊断标准

1 西医诊断标准及分型

在国际头痛协会（IHS）2013 年发表的 ICHD–3 的试用版[17]中，由于偏头痛分类复杂，以及本《指南》的推荐方案主要针对先兆偏头痛和无先兆偏头痛，因此本《指南》仅介绍此两型诊断标准，其他偏头痛诊断可参考 ICHD–3。

1.1 无先兆偏头痛

①至少有 5 次满足以下②～④的头痛发作。

②头痛发作持续 4～72 小时（未经治疗或治疗无效）。

③头痛至少具有下列 4 项特征中的 2 项：偏侧分布；搏动性；疼痛程度为中或重度；因上楼梯或其他类似日常躯体活动而加重。日常活动导致头痛加重或头痛导致日常活动受限（如走路或登楼）。

④头痛发作时至少具有下列症状中的 1 项：恶心和（或）呕吐；畏光和（或）畏声。

⑤无法用另一种 ICHD–3 的头痛疾患诊断来更好地解释。

1.2 先兆偏头痛

①至少有 2 次符合以下②和③的发作。

②以下 1 种或多种完全可逆的先兆症状：视觉；感觉；言语和（或）语言；运动；脑干；视网膜。

③下列 4 项特征中至少有 2 项：至少 1 种先兆症状逐渐进展≥5 分钟和（或）两种或多种症状相继出现；每个先兆症状持续 5～60 分钟；至少 1 个先兆症状是单侧的；先兆伴随头痛或在先兆发生 60 分钟内发生头痛。

④没有另一个 ICHD–3 的头痛疾患诊断能更好地解释，且短暂性缺血发作已被排除。

2 中医诊断标准及分型

2.1 中医诊断标准

根据 1994 年国家中医药管理局制定的《中医病证诊断疗效标准》[18]中"头风诊断依据"，偏头痛中医诊断依据如下：

①头痛部位多在头部一侧额颞、前额、颠顶，或左或右辗转发作，或呈全头痛。头痛的性质多为跳痛、刺痛、胀痛、昏痛、隐痛，或头痛如裂等。头痛每次发作可持续数分钟、数小时、数天，也有持续数周者。

②隐袭起病，逐渐加重或反复发作。

③应查血常规，测血压，必要时做腰穿、骨穿，脑电图。有条件时做经颅多普勒、CT、磁共振等检查，以明确头痛的病因，排除器质性疾病。

2.2 中医辨证分型标准

2.2.1 经脉辨证

根据邱茂良第 5 版《针灸学》[19]及郭霭春《黄帝内经灵枢校注语译》[20]确定偏头痛常见的经脉辨证类型：

少阳经症状：头痛部位以一侧或两侧侧头为主，集中于外眼角周围；可伴口苦，叹气，汗出，面色少华，耳部、咽喉、面颊不适，胸胁部疼痛，侧面躯体不适等。

阳明经症状：头痛部位以一侧或者两侧前额为主；可伴恶心呕吐，胃肠不适等。

太阳经症状：头痛部位以后头、项部为主；可伴目痛，见风流泪、鼻塞多涕、项背部本经循行部位疼痛等。

厥阴经症状：头痛部位以头顶为主。可伴心慌胸闷，情志异常，手心热等。

2.2.2 其他辨证

根据 2002 年中华人民共和国卫生部制定发布的《中药新药临床研究指导原则》[21] 中 "中药新药治疗偏头痛的临床研究指导原则"，确定中医辨证分型如下：

2.2.2.1 肝阳上亢型

主症：头痛而胀，心烦易怒，目赤，口苦。

次症：面红，口干，舌红，苔黄，脉弦或弦数。

2.2.2.2 痰浊型

主症：头痛如裹，胸脘满闷，呕恶痰涎。

次症：口淡，食少，舌胖大，舌苔白腻，脉弦滑。

2.2.2.3 肾虚型

主症：头痛而空，眩晕，腰酸膝软，五心烦热。

次症：神疲乏力，耳鸣，舌质红，少苔，脉沉细无力。

2.2.2.4 瘀血型

主症：头痛如刺，经久不愈，固定不移。

次症：舌质紫暗，或有瘀斑、瘀点，苔薄白，脉沉细或细涩。

2.2.2.5 气血亏虚型

主症：头痛隐隐反复发作，遇劳加重。

次症：心悸，食少纳呆，自汗，气短，神疲乏力，面色苍白，舌质淡，苔薄白，脉沉细而弱。

针灸治疗概况

1 现代文献

1.1 辨证治疗方面

针灸治疗可以在偏头痛发生的各个时期进行。在头痛发作期，遵循中医理论中的"急则治其标"观念，临床重视透穴刺法，多采用放血、电针等较强的刺激以行气活血通络，从而获得迅速、明显的即时镇痛效果。在头痛缓解期，往往遵循中医"缓则治其本""标本同治"的理论，多采用较发作期轻的刺激，两次治疗之间的间隔时间较头痛发作期长，可获得较好的近期及远期疗效，对预防头痛的发作也有良好效果。其中使用频率较高的是以下几组腧穴：①局部：阿是穴、丝竹空配率谷、太阳配风池、颔厌至悬厘连线（颔厌、悬颅、悬厘）、头临泣至承灵连线（头临泣、目窗、正营、承灵）；②远端：合谷、列缺、太冲、足临泣、丘墟、阳陵泉；③耳穴：神门、额、颞、枕、交感、脑点。

1.2 刺灸法方面

近20年的针灸治疗偏头痛文献主要涉及以下几种疗法：针刺、电针、放血、耳穴、火针、穴位注射、皮肤针、刮痧等，可单独或相互组合进行综合治疗。

2 古代文献

古代针灸治疗偏头痛主要有针刺、艾灸、放血、刮痧四种疗法。其中，针法最为常用，以少阳经穴局部取穴为主，配合远端取穴，常用的有颔厌、风池、悬厘、悬颅、丝竹空、后顶、头维、正营等，远端选取列缺、合谷。灸法取穴也以局部配合远端取穴，穴位同针刺法。放血疗法主要以局部取穴为主，常用太阳紫脉、百会。刮痧主要采用局部取穴。

3 名医经验

现代名医家治疗偏头痛，多在经络辨证基础上，结合病因、气血津液及脏腑辨证，以局部取穴为主，灵活配合远端辨证选穴。在刺灸法上，以针刺为主，还涉及放血、耳穴压丸、火针等疗法。

针灸治疗和推荐方案

1 针灸治疗的原则及特点

1.1 针灸治疗原则

治疗原则[22,23]：行气活血、疏通少阳为主。发作期通络止痛、辨经论治为主；缓解期疏通经络，配合辨证论治、综合各种针灸疗法。

取穴原则：发作期以少阳经穴、阿是穴为主，配合辨经取穴及耳穴。缓解期在发作期取穴基础上结合辨证配穴。

1.2 针灸治疗特点

针灸治疗可以在偏头痛发生的各个时期进行。在头痛发作期，遵循中医理论中的"急则治其标"观念。临床重视透穴刺法，多采用放血、电针等较强的刺激以行气活血通络，从而获得迅速、明显的即时镇痛效果。在头痛缓解期，往往遵循中医"缓则治其本""标本同治"的理论，多采用较发作期轻的刺激，两次治疗之间的间隔时间较头痛发作期长，可获得较好的近期及远期疗效，对预防头痛的发作也有良好效果。

2 主要结局指标

头痛缓解时间（发作期）。

头痛天数/月。

头痛发作次数/月。

疼痛强度：视觉模拟评分法（VAS）。

头痛复发人数/24 小时（发作期）。

头痛时间（h）/月。

用药人数。

头痛指数。

McGill 疼痛问卷量表（MPQ）评分。

偏头痛残疾程度评估问卷（MIDAS）评分。

3 注意事项[19]

3.1 操作注意事项

患者在过于饥饿、疲劳、精神紧张、情绪激动情况下，不宜立即进行针刺治疗。对身体瘦弱、气血亏虚的患者，应取卧位。针刺手法不宜过重。

临床操作常见的晕针现象、皮下血肿及气肿、滞针、弯针、断针以及气胸等意外情况出现时应根据病情轻重给予对症处理。

为患者做好健康指导，讲解针灸治疗偏头痛的机制、疗法及注意事项，使患者心中有数，树立治疗信心。

3.2 禁忌证

孕妇：妇女怀孕 3 个月以内者，下腹部禁针；怀孕 3 个月以上者，腹部及腰骶部不宜针刺。三阴交、合谷等穴有通经活血作用，孕妇禁针；对有习惯性流产史者，尤须慎重。

病灶局部：有皮肤感染溃疡、瘢痕或肿瘤的部位不宜针灸。

出血性疾病：常有自发性出血或凝血障碍的患者不宜针灸。

合并重病：合并心脑血管、肝、肾、造血系统等严重疾病以及精神病患者不宜针灸。

4 患者自我护理

饮食护理：天气转冷时，注意冷暖，注意增减衣物，尤应注意颈部保暖。治疗期间，多吃水果、蔬菜和营养丰富易消化的食物；禁食肥甘厚腻、生痰助湿的食物；禁食生冷刺激性食物；禁食海鲜、虾等食物。

生活起居护理：治疗期间尽量避免感冒；睡眠要充足，每晚保证 7 ~ 8 小时睡眠，避免收看紧张和刺激性强的影视节目。

心理护理：注意维护患者良好的心态，避免其情绪过于激动、烦躁或悲伤忧郁。

5 推荐方案

5.1 发作期

5.1.1 放血

放血具有活血泻热、通络止痛之功，特别适用于发作期正邪交争的阶段；实验研究证实刺破体表的微细体液管道，可起到刺激和调整微循环的功能状态的作用[24]，具有起效快、治疗时间短、效果显著等优点。

取穴：①局部刺血：局部压痛点或太阳穴周围浅表络脉。②耳郭刺血：主穴：耳尖，耳轮络脉或耳背上 1/3 有血管充盈处（有则取）；配穴：颞（枕）、胰胆、神门、交感、皮质下、内分泌穴。

针刺方法：针具：三棱针。手法：①局部刺血：皮肤常规消毒后，左手拇、食指固定穴位周围皮肤，右手持三棱针点刺出血，挤血同时用 75% 酒精棉球擦拭局部，点刺放出适量血液或黏液后用无菌干棉球或棉签擦拭或按压。②耳郭刺血：耳尖、耳轮络脉、耳背上 1/3 血管充盈处按摩 1 ~ 3 分钟，使明显充血，医者用左手拇指、示指和中指固定耳郭，局部常规消毒后用三棱针点刺出血，出血数滴。其余耳穴：局部常规消毒后，三棱针点刺，使之呈轻微点状出血，点刺放出适量血液或黏液后用无菌干棉球或棉签擦拭或按压。

注意事项：①每次刺血穴位不宜过多，且所选穴位不宜过于分散，应当集中在痛处及周围；②放血当日，针孔处注意避水；③注意血压、心率变化，注意晕针或晕血的发生；④本法配合常规针法使用；⑤缓解期肝阳上亢型、瘀血型患者也可参照使用，治疗频率为 1 周 1 次。

『推荐』

> 推荐建议：发作期偏头痛推荐首先使用局部刺络，耳轮或耳背上 1/3 有络脉或者全身症状明显者可同时配合耳郭刺血。缓解期肝阳上亢型、瘀血型患者也可参照治疗。[GRADE 1D]

解释：本《指南》小组共纳入相关现代文献 4 篇[25 - 28]，经综合分析，形成证据体发现，局部刺络配合耳穴刺络可降低头痛发作频率、治疗无效率、头痛积分、头痛指数，缩短发作时间等。证据体质量等级经 GRADE 评价后，因其纳入文献设计质量、精确性不高，并存在发表偏倚，最终证据体质量等级为低或极低。但综合利弊平衡、患者意愿、资源消耗与成本分析及专家意见共识，并结合临床实际，仍然对本治疗方案进行强推荐。

5.1.2 毫针刺法（电针）

针刺具有行气活血、通络止痛的作用，适用于发作期、缓解期各个阶段；实验研究证明：针刺能调节支配血管的自主神经，改善脑血管异常的舒缩状态，使微循环获得改善，减少炎性和致痛物质的渗出，以达到预防和缓解疼痛的效果。具有疗效好、操作方便、辅助作用少等优点。

取穴：①穴方一：主穴：阿是穴、丝竹空、率谷、太阳、风池、合谷、太冲、足临泣。配穴：阳陵泉、外关。②穴方二：主穴：对侧顶颞后斜线下 2/5、双侧顶旁 2 线。配穴：额颞部痛配同侧率谷，头顶痛配同侧风池。在上述二方基础上，兼有厥阴经症状者：加内关、人中、神门、百会；兼有阳明经症状者：加头维；兼有膀胱经症状者：加天柱。上述腧穴中，局部腧穴取患侧，远端腧穴取双侧。

针刺方法：患者取坐位或仰卧位，选用直径 0.30mm、长度 40mm 的毫针；穴方一中的阿是穴，选 1~2 个为宜。若疼痛是从一点渐及周围，此点即为针刺部位；若疼痛区域固定，则选痛区中心位置为针刺部位；若疼痛面积较大，无法定位，则通过寻按痛区，找到明显压痛点或头皮肿胀点，以此为针刺部位，上下小幅度提插；丝竹空、率谷相对进针后平刺 1.5~2 寸，相互透刺，行小幅度快频率捻转；余穴针刺得气后，行提插捻转平补平泻法；各行针 1 分钟。阿是穴接电针仪，使用疏密波，频率为 2~100Hz，刺激强度以病人能耐受为度，余穴每隔 10 分钟行针 1 次。头部取穴以患侧为主，远端穴位双侧取穴。穴方二中头针操作，用平刺快速进针，用小幅度快频率捻转，行针 2 分钟，每 10 分钟行针 1 次。

疗程：每次留针 30 分钟，头针可留至 1 小时。治疗频率隔日 1 次，10 次为 1 个疗程。

『推荐』

> 推荐建议：发作期偏头痛推荐以少阳经穴为主，配合经络辨证取穴，可用透穴针刺结合阿是穴电针治疗。［GRADE 1BCD］

解释：本《指南》小组共纳入相关现代文献 19 篇[29-47]，经综合分析，形成证据体发现，少阳经穴为主配合辨经针刺治疗可缓解头痛强度，降低治疗无效率，减少用药，提高生活质量等。证据体质量等级经 GRADE 评价后，因其纳入文献设计质量、一致性、精确性差别较大，且存在发表偏倚，最终证据体质量等级分中、低、极低。但综合利弊平衡、患者意愿、资源消耗与成本分析及专家意见共识，并结合临床实际，仍然对于本治疗方案进行强推荐。

5.1.3 火针

火针借火热之力直接激发经气，能鼓舞气血运行，达到通络止痛之功；另一方面亦使瘀血等有形之邪，随针孔直接排出体外，以达开门祛邪之效；实验研究证实其能使病变局部的温度升高，微循环的血流加快，血流状态明显好转[48]。具有治疗时间短、治疗次数少、每次治疗间隔时间较长的优点。

取穴：阿是穴、头维（患侧）、率谷（患侧）。

针刺方法：穴位常规消毒，采用中号火针，将针身的前中段烧至通红，对准阿是穴、患侧头维及率谷穴迅速刺入 0.2~0.3 寸并拔出，出针后用消毒干棉球按压针孔片刻。

注意事项：①火针治疗当日，针孔处注意避水；②针刺要避开动脉及神经干，勿损伤内脏和重要器官。

『推荐』

> 推荐建议：发作期偏头痛在针刺治疗基础上，可配合使用火针疗法。［GRADE 2D］

解释：本《指南》小组共纳入相关现代文献 1 篇[49]，经分析，火针可降低治疗无效率，减轻头痛强度。证据体质量等级经 GRADE 评价后，因其纳入文献设计质量、精确性不高，并存在发表偏倚，最终证据体质量等级为极低。但综合利弊平衡、患者意愿、资源消耗与成本分析及专家意见共识，并结合临床实际，对于本治疗方案进行弱推荐。

5.2 缓解期

缓解期可进行针灸综合治疗，该疗法安全有效，且其具有因人而异、操作较为简便、疗效显著、痛苦较小等优点。针刺治疗与西医预防性药物治疗的疗效进行比较的临床研究显示：针刺的预防性作用至少与药物作用相当，但针刺的副作用却明显少于药物[50]。

取穴：在发作期毫针刺法（电针）方案基础上结合脏腑、津液气血辨证。

肝阳上亢型：加颔厌透悬颅、列缺、太溪、行间。

痰浊型：加颔厌透悬颅、列缺、丰隆、内关。

瘀血型：加膈俞、血海、足三里、三阴交。

肾虚、气血不足型：加足三里、气海、三阴交、太溪、肾俞。

上述腧穴中，局部腧穴取患侧，远端腧穴取双侧。

针刺方法：主穴毫针刺法见发作期操作部分。余穴针刺得气后，行提插捻转平补平泻法。每隔 10 分钟行针 1 次。肝阳上亢型患者可结合耳尖、耳轮放血；瘀血型患者可结合痛点或太阳紫脉放血；肾虚、气血不足型每次取 2~4 穴，施温针灸，每穴 3 壮。

疗程：每次留针 30 分钟，头针可留至 1 小时。治疗频率隔日 1 次，10 次为 1 个疗程。放血可根据患者情况 1 周 1~2 次。

『推荐』

> 推荐建议：缓解期偏头痛推荐以少阳经穴为主，兼顾经络、脏腑辨证取穴的毫针刺法，同时可配合头针、电针、温针灸、放血。[GRADE 1BCD]

解释：本《指南》小组共纳入相关现代文献 20 篇[29-47,51]，经综合分析，形成证据体发现，以少阳经穴为主兼顾辨经辨证毫针刺，并配合头针、电针、温针灸、放血等综合治疗可缓解头痛强度，降低治疗无效率、头痛发作次数、头痛积分，缩短头痛时间，减少用药，提高生活质量等。证据体质量等级经 GRADE 评价后，因其纳入文献设计质量、一致性、精确性差别较大，且存在发表偏倚，最终证据体质量等级分中、低、极低。但综合利弊平衡、患者意愿、资源消耗与成本分析及专家意见共识，并结合临床实际，仍然对本治疗方案进行强推荐。

参考文献

[1] 步怀恩，王建华，王泓午. 偏头痛流行病学特点 [J]. 天津中医药大学学报，2006，25 (2)：82.

[2] 张秀峰，边建超. 偏头痛的遗传流行病学研究进展 [J]. 国外医学·遗传学分册，2005，28 (1)：41 – 45.

[3] 赵英. 偏头痛的流行病学特点 [J]. 中国社区医生，2005，21 (11)：9 – 10.

[4] Yu S, Liu R, Z Getal. The prevalence and burden of primary headaches in China：A population – based door – to – door survey [J]. Headache, 2012, 52 (4)：528 – 591.

[5] Bartleson JD, Cutrer FM. Migraine update, diagnosis and treatment [J]. Minn Med, 2010, 93 (5)：36 – 41.

[6] Piane M, Lullt P, Farinellt I, et al. Genetics of migratine and pharmacogenomics：some considerations [J]. Headache and pain, 2007, 8 (6)：334 – 339.

[7] Lay Cl, Broner Sw. Migraine in women [J]. Neurologic clinics, 2009, 27 (2)：503 – 511.

[8] Stovner LJ, Zwart Ja, Hagen K, et al. Epidemiology of headache in Europe [J]. Neurology, 2006, 13 (4)：333 – 45.

[9] Gutman, Sharon A. Quick reference neuroscience for rehabilitation professionals：The essential neurologic principles underlying rehabilitation practice 2nd. Thorofare [M], NJ：Slack, 2008.

[10] 中华医学会疼痛学分会头面痛学组. 中国偏头痛诊断治疗指南 [J]. 中国疼痛医学杂志，2011，17 (2)：65 – 85.

[11] Aminoff, Roger P. Simon, David A. Greenberg, et al. Clinical neurology 7th ed [M]. New York：Lange medical books/ Mcgrew – Hill, 2009.

[12] Rossi P, Ambrosini A, Buzzl MG. Prodroms and predictorsof migratine attack [J]. Functional neurology, 2005, 20 (4)：185 – 191.

[13] Samuels, Allan H. Popper, Martin A. Adams and victor's principles of neurology 9th ed [M]. New York：Mcgraw – Hill medical, 2009：chapter10.

[14] Tintinalli, Judith E. Emergency medicine：A comprehensive study guide [emergency medicine (tintinall)] [M]. New York：Mcgraw – Hill Companies, 2010.

[15] Bigal Me, Arruda Ma. Migratine in the prediatric population – evolving concepts [J]. Headache. 2010, 50 (7)：1130 – 1143.

[16] Dalessio, Stephen D. Silberstein, Richard B. Lipton, et al. Wolff's Headache and other head pain. 7th ed [M]. Oxford：Oxford university press, 2001.

[17] Headache classification committee of the international headache society (IHS). The international classification of headache disorders. 3rd edition (beta version). Cephalagta, 2012, 33：629 – 808.

[18] 国家中医药管理局. 中医病证诊断疗效标准 [M]. 南京：南京大学出版社，1994：145 – 147.

[19] 邱茂良. 针灸学 [M]. 上海：上海科学技术出版社，1985.

[20] 郭霭春. 黄帝内经灵枢校注语译 [M]. 天津. 天津科学技术出版社，1999.

[21] 郑筱萸. 中药新药临床研究指导原则（2002 试行版）[M]. 北京：中国医药科技出版社，2002：106.

[22] Melchart D, Thormaehlen J, Hager S. Acupuncture versus placebo versus sumatriptan for early treat-

ment of migatine attacks：A randomized controlled trial ［J］．Intern med，2003，253（2）：181 -188.

[23] 艾民，常亚娟，张洋，等．针刺双侧太阳、风池穴治疗偏头痛的疗效观察 ［J］．针灸临床杂志，2011，27（9）：9 -10.

[24] 黄美惠．以头部刺血疗法为主治疗偏头痛的临床研究 ［D］．广东中医药大学，2012：56.

[25] 王非，孙海东．刺络放血疗法治疗偏头痛94 例 ［J］．中医外治杂志，2010，19（5）：42 -43.

[26] 李华贵，曹晓滨．三棱针点刺阿是穴治疗偏头痛疗效观察 ［J］．新疆医科大学学报，2009，32（7）：861 -863.

[27] 佟波．放血疗法治疗偏头痛35 例临床观察 ［J］．中国民康医学，2013，25（16）：52.

[28] 单秋华．耳穴综合疗法治疗发作期普通偏头痛即刻疗效观察 ［J］．山东中医药大学学报，2006，30（3）：201 -203.

[29] 李桂敏，严伟，殷建权．针刺治疗偏头痛急性发作疗效观察 ［J］．上海针灸杂志，2010，29（7）：439 -441.

[30] 蔡玉颖．透穴刺法治疗偏头痛的临床疗效及对脑血流速度的影响 ［J］．中国针灸，2006，（26）：177 -179.

[31] 李甘．电针预防性治疗偏头痛的临床观察 ［D］．湖北中医药大学，2013：5 -6.

[32] 郑盛惠，吴玉娟，焦建凯，等．赤凤迎源针法治疗偏头痛临床疗效及对脑血流速度的影响 ［J］．针灸临床杂志，2013，29（6）：45 -48.

[33] 宋文博．以风池穴为主针刺治疗偏头痛的临床研究 ［D］．黑龙江中医药大学，2010：33.

[34] Linde K，Streng A，Jurgens S，et al. Acupuncture for patents with migraine：A randomized controlled trial ［J］．Jama，2005，293（17）：2118 -2125.

[35] Streng A，Linde K，Hoppe A，et al. Effectiveness and tolerability of acupuncture compared with metoprolol in migraine prophylaxis ［J］．Headache，2006，46（10）：1492 -1502.

[36] Allatis G，De Lorenzo C，Quirico Pe，et al. Non - pharmacological approaches to chronic headaches：Transcutaneous electrical nerve stimulation，Lasertherapy and acupuncture in transformed migraine treatment ［J］．Neurol SCI，2003，（Suppl2）：S138 -142.

[37] 杨雄庆．针刺对偏头痛的临床疗效观察 ［J］．浙江中医药大学学报，2013，37（5）：617 -619.

[38] 李琛．针刺治疗偏头痛39 例疗效观察 ［J］．临床合理用药，2011，4（11A）：153.

[39] 祝坤平．针刺治疗偏头痛45 例临床体会 ［J］．航空航天医学杂志，2011，22（9）：1147 -1148.

[40] Ting Li，Hui Zheng，Clatdia M. Witt，et. al. Acupuncture for migraine prophylaxis - a randomized trial. CMAJ，2012. DOI：10. 1503/CMAJ. 110551.

[41] Gianni Allais，Cristina De Lorenzo，Piero E. Quirico，et al. Acupuncture in the prophylactic treatment of migraine. Headache，2002，42：855 -861/CMAJ. 110551.

[42] C - P Yang. Acupuncture versus topiramate in chronic migraine prophylaxis a randomized clinical trial ［J］．Cephalalgia，2011，31（15）：1510 -1521.

[43] Aldo Liguori，Filomena Petti，Alfio Bangrazi. Comparison of pharmacological treatment versus acupuncture treatment for migraine without aura - analysis of socio - medical parameters ［J］．Journal of traditional Chinese medicine，2000，20（3）：231 -240.

[44] Andrea Streng，Klaus Linde，Andrea Hoppe. Effectiveness and tolerability of acupuncture compared with metoprolol in migraine prophylaxis ［J］．Headache，2006，（12）：1492 -2006.

[45] Lin Peng Wang, Hui Lin Liu, Cun Zhi Liu. Efficacy of acupuncture for migraine prophylaxis [J]. Pain, 2011 (152): 1864 - 1871.

[46] Jorge Vas, Inmaculada Aguilar. Study protocol for a pragmatic randomized controlled trial [J], BMC Complementary and Alternative Medicine, 2008, (8): 12.

[47] 赵丽君. 运动头针治疗偏头痛 50 例 [J]. 中国中医药信息杂志, 2002, 9 (11): 64.

[48] 崔芮, 盛丽. 贺氏针灸三通法 [M]. 北京: 中国医药科技出版社, 1995.

[49] 林国华, 范兆金, 李丽霞, 等. 火针与电针治疗偏头痛的临床对照研究 [J]. 新中医, 2001, 33 (8): 43 - 44.

[50] Linde K, Al; ais G, Brinkhaus B, Etal. Acupuncture for migraine prophylaxis [DB/CD]. Cochrane database syst rev, 2009, (1): CD001218.

[51] 朱国祥. 温针灸结合叩刺法治疗偏头痛瘀血型 79 例疗效观察 [J]. 针灸临床杂志, 1999, 15 (5): 40 - 41.

附 录

1 本《指南》专家组成员和编写组成员

专家组成员

姓名	性别	职称	工作单位	课题中的分工
杨金洪	女	主任医师	中国中医科学院针灸研究所	组织及协调任务分配
魏庆兴	男	主任医师	中国中医科学院针灸研究所	审核临床问题、确定推荐方案
刘家瑛	女	主任医师	中国中医科学院针灸研究所	审核临床问题、确定推荐方案
姜爱萍	女	主任医师	中国中医科学院针灸研究所	审核临床问题、确定推荐方案
曹建萍	女	副主任医师	中国中医科学院针灸研究所	审核临床问题、确定推荐方案
费宇彤	女	循证医学	北京中医药大学循证医学中心	《指南》方法指导
张早华	男	研究员	中国中医科学院信息所	文献检索、质量评价方法指导
王思成	男	主任科员	国家中医药管理局科技司	政策指导
张咏梅	女	副译审	中国中医科学院	《指南》英文版校对审核
王惠珠	女	正译审	中国中医科学院针灸研究所	《指南》英文版校对审核

编写组成员

	姓名	性别	学历/职称	工作单位	课题中的分工
组长	吴中朝	男	博士 主任医师	中国中医科学院针灸研究所	总负责人，管理、组织《指南》的编写以及分配任务
组员	王京京	女	副主任医师	中国中医科学院针灸研究所	副总负责人，组织《指南》的撰写及分配任务，收集临床关注问题，评价英文文献，起草、修改《指南》
	胡 静	女	硕士 主治医师	中国中医科学院针灸研究所	检索、评价文献，收集临床关注问题，起草、修改、完善《指南》，专家意见咨询，《指南》英文版翻译
	焦 玥	女	硕士 主治医师	中国中医科学院针灸研究所	检索、评价文献，收集临床关注问题，起草、修改、完善《指南》，专家意见咨询，《指南》英文版翻译
	周文娜	女	硕士研究生	中国中医科学院针灸研究所	文献评估、专家意见咨询
	黄子明	男	硕士	中国中医科学院针灸研究所	评价英文文献，《指南》英文版翻译
	王丽娜	女	硕士 住院医师	宝鸡中医院	《指南》英文版翻译
	郭宇鹏	女	博士	中国中医科学院针灸研究所	《指南》英文版翻译
	陈仲杰	女	博士 主治医师	中国中医科学院针灸研究所	《指南》英文版翻译
	李荣俊	男	硕士 住院医师	中国中医科学院针灸研究所	修改《指南》

2 临床问题

2.1 医生关注问题

问卷从偏头痛的定义到卫生经济学共设 18 个问题，每问题根据关注等级分别给予 0~4 分，将每一问题总的分数汇总后，按照关注度从高到低将问题列举如下（共 39 份）：

具体操作方法。（138）

疗效。（131）

针灸干预时机。（125）

取穴。（124）

危险因素、潜在的诱发因素。（121）

治疗间隔时间（或频次）。（119）

辨证分型。（118）

诊断。（113）

预后。（109）

各种注意事项。（108）

合并其他疗法的适应证及方法选择。（105）

支持以上结论的证据级别及推荐方案。（104）

偏头痛定义。（102）

病因病机。（102）

分型。（97）

病人耐受度。（93）

不良反应。（92）

卫生经济学评价。（80）

此外，在开放题中涉及以下几个问题：

偏头痛的心理学观察。（2）

因患者的性别、年龄、病程的不同在治疗上的差异。（2）

实用性及可操作性。（2）

西医检查手段及诊断方法。（1）

病史、家族史。

针、灸应分开论述。

综合应用时，针灸应当在西药之前还是之后用。

怎样保证中医药治疗偏头痛疗效的确切以致可以在全世界尤其是在欧洲进行推广？

针灸临床试验中如何应用盲法？

在网络上查找指南的方法。

2.2 患者关注问题

问卷从偏头痛的症状到预后共设施 15 个问题，每问题后设"是""否"两个选项，统计时只考虑"是"的频率，以确定关注度。按照关注度从高到低将问题列举如下：（共 18 份）

偏头痛的潜在诱发因素或危险因素。（18）

偏头痛的疼痛发作时应如何处理。（18）

针灸治疗偏头痛的疗程为多长时间？（18）

自我护理要点。（17）

针灸治疗最佳时机。（17）

针灸治疗偏头痛是否有效？（16）

针灸治疗偏头痛的疗效等达到多少？（15）

有哪些合并治疗措施、是否需要合并治疗？（15）

针灸治疗偏头痛的预后。（15）

偏头痛的主要症状。（14）

偏头痛的主要病因及病变机理。（14）

两次针灸的间隔时间多长？（14）

能否耐受针灸治疗？（14）

针灸治疗是否安全？（13）

针灸治疗的不良反应有哪些？（13）

此外，在开放题中涉及以下几个问题：

用什么样的针灸方法最快最好？

针灸治疗同时，还需同时服用什么药物？

一次针灸治疗的时间是多长？

偏头痛是否有遗传性，致病因素是什么，各种不同针灸治疗方法之间的区别。

药物和针灸哪一个治疗效果更好？

合并眼痛、牙痛的偏头痛是否需要更长的治疗时间？

针灸治疗偏头痛的疗效如何，能否根除？

3 疗效评价指标的分级

疗效评价指标	综合评级
头痛缓解时间（急性期）	9
头痛天数/月	9
头痛发作次数/月	9
头痛强度（VAS）/月	9
头痛复发人数/24 小时（急性期）	8
头痛时间（h）/月	8
用药人数	8
头痛指数	8
McGill 疼痛问卷量表（MPQ）评分	7
偏头痛残疾程度评估问卷（MIDAS）评分	7
健康调查简表（SF-36）	6
偏头痛生活质量量表（MSQ）评分	6
不良反应发生率	5
中医证候积分	4
无效率（尼莫地平法）	4
TCD 各动脉血流速	3
5-HT	2
NO	2

4 检索范围、检索策略及结果

4.1 检索范围

根据偏头痛的特点和文献特点由编写组确定《指南》文献检索的纳入标准和排除标准。由编写组根据临床问题分别确定现代文献、古代文献和名医家经验检索策略。检索策略包括检索词、检索工具、检索范围等。

检索策略由流行病学专家和临床专家审核通过。

4.1.1 现代文献检索策略和方法

由编写组在文献专家指导下，确定现代文献检索词、检索式和检索范围。检索文献范围包括中文文献、英文文献。

由编写组根据确定的文献检索策略，采用电子检索和手工检索结合的形式进行检索。

4.1.2 古代文献检索策略和方法

由编写组根据疾病特点确定古代文献检索词、古代文献检索数据库、书目及相关版本。

4.1.3 名医家经验检索策略和方法

由编写组根据偏头痛特点确定名医家经验检索词和检索书目。由2名起草组人员采用手工检索的方法对每个书目进行检索，查找符合纳入标准的条目。

4.2 检索策略

4.2.1 中文现代文献检索方法

在检索中文现代文献过程中，为防止漏检及尽量减少重复，我们进行了预检索，以确定最终的检索关键词及检索方法，最终确定现代文献检索策略如下：在中国生物医学文献光盘数据库（CBM，1994～2013）、中文生物医学期刊全文数据库（CMCC，1994～2013）以及CNKI（1979～2013）中对中文现代文献进行检索。同时收集未发表的文献（包括针灸学会会议论文、研究生及博士生论文等相关的汇编等）。以"偏头痛"为关键词进行检索，在检索结果中以"针刺/针灸/电针/耳穴/耳压/耳豆/耳针/皮肤针/梅花针/七星针/三棱针/刺络/放血/刺络放血/刺血/灸法/艾灸/灸/头针/头皮针/穴位注射/水针/穴位埋线/火针/刮痧/拔罐/火罐/针罐"为或然检索词进行再检索。

4.2.2 英文现代文献检索方法

英文现代文献委托解放军医学图书馆数据库中心进行检索并下载。以"randomized controlled trial and migraine and acupuncture / electroacupuncture / moxibustion / cupping / auricular acupuncture / acupressure and ear / cutaneous acupuncture"为关键词在MEDLINE、EMBASE数据库检索国外文献。

4.2.3 日、韩文现代文献检索方法

日、韩文现代文献委托中国中医科学院信息所检索。

日文文献以"acupuncture""migraine"为关键词，在medical online数据库中进行检索。韩文文献以"acupuncture""migraine"为关键词，在韩国医学论文数据库（Korean Medical Database）中进行检索。

4.2.4 古代文献检索方法

检索来源：数据库检索——中华医典。

　　　　　手工检索——中国中医科学院图书馆。

检索关键字：偏头风、偏头痛/疼、偏正头风、偏正头痛/疼、头半寒（痛/疼）、半边头痛/疼、头偏痛/疼、头项偏痛/疼、头风偏痛/疼、半边头风。

检索方法及过程：在中华医典中分别以"偏头风""偏头痛/疼""偏正头风""偏正头痛/疼""头半寒（痛/疼）""半边头痛/疼""头偏痛/疼""头项偏痛/疼""头风偏痛/疼""半边头风"为关键词进行检索。

在《中国中医科学院图书馆馆藏古籍书目》中对相关古籍进行检索，查询其检书号，并参考文献专家意见对其版本进行选择和记录。

在中国中医科学院图书馆古籍阅览室对检出文献进行核查工作，确定最终检出文献的数量及准确性。

4.3 检索结果

检索文献：458篇。

排除重复检索及重复发表文献、动物实验、文献研究、文献综述、科普性文章等，新纳入文献195篇。

原有文献8篇。

其中，SR 3 篇（均为新纳入），RCT 38 篇（新纳入 35 篇，原有 3 篇），观察性 162 篇（新纳入 157 篇，原有 5 篇）。

4.3.1 古代医籍纳入文献

共检索到 25 部古代医籍中与偏头风的针灸治疗相关的条目 151 条，符合偏头痛的特点。

序号	专著	序号	专著
1	《备急千金要方》	14	《医经小学》
2	《外台秘要》	15	《奇效良方》
3	《针灸甲乙经》	16	《医学入门》
4	《铜人腧穴针灸图经》	17	《针灸大全》
5	《圣济总录》	18	《东医宝鉴》
6	《太平圣惠方》	19	《普济方》
7	《西方子明堂灸经》	20	《针灸节要聚英》
8	《琼瑶神书》	21	《针灸大成》
9	《针灸资生经》	22	《针方六集》
10	《针灸集书》	23	《类经图翼》
11	《循经考穴编》	24	《针灸逢源》
12	《扁鹊神应针灸玉龙经》	25	《针灸易学》
13	《神应经》		

4.3.2 近现代医籍纳入文献（共 43 部）

	主编	著作名	出处
1	承淡安	《承淡安针灸师承录》	头痛（第 154 页）
2	项 平	《承淡安针灸经验集》	神经系统和精神疾病（第 243 页）
3	承为奋	《承淡安针灸选集》	头痛（第 101 页）
4	承淡安	《中国针灸学》	偏头痛（第 266 页）
5	俞中元	《中国百年百名中医临床家丛书·承淡安》	头部门（第 97 页）
6	陆瘦燕	《金针实验录》	头痛（第 63 页）
7	陆焱垚	《针灸名家陆瘦燕学术经验集》	偏头痛（第 3 页）
8	朱 琏	《新针灸学》	偏头痛（第 206 页）
9	鲁之俊	《新编针灸学》	偏头痛（第 72 页）
10	杨甲三	《杨甲三临证论治》	头痛（第 92 页）
11	胡 慧	《杨甲三》	头痛（第 26 页）
12	邱茂良	《针灸学》	头痛（第 215 页）
13	贺普仁	《针灸三通法操作图解》	头痛（第 58、238、355、489 页）
14	贺普仁	《针灸治痛》	头痛（第 28 页）
15	贺普仁	《针灸三通法临床应用》	偏头痛（第 70 页）

	主编	著作名	出处
16	贺普仁	《火针疗法图解（贺氏针灸三通法之一）》	头痛（第58页）
17	贺普仁	《毫针疗法图解（贺氏针灸三通法之二）》	头痛（第51页）
18	贺普仁	《三棱针疗法图解（贺氏针灸三通法之三）》	头痛（第28页）
19	贺普仁	《针灸歌赋临床应用》	头痛（第175页）
20	佘靖	《中国现代百名中医临床家丛书·贺普仁》	偏头痛（第155页）
21	程莘农	《中医学问答题库·针灸学》	头痛（第85页）
22	程莘农	《中国针灸学》	头痛（第530页）
23	郑魁山	《郑氏针灸全集》	偏头痛（第644页）
24	郑魁山	《针灸临证经验集》	偏头痛（第248页）
25	郑魁山	《针灸集锦》	头痛（第361页）
26	王雪苔	《中国针灸大全》	头痛（第62页）
27	焦顺发	《中国针灸学术真传》	偏头痛（第189页）
28	石学敏	《针灸学》	偏头痛（第204页）
29	石学敏	《石学敏针灸全集》	头痛（第377页）
30	石学敏	《针灸推拿学》	头痛（第255页）
31	石学敏	《中国针灸奇术》	偏头痛（第348页）
32	石学敏	《常见病实用针灸配方》	头痛（第69页）
33	石学敏	《中医针灸临床手册》	头痛（第281页）
34	石学敏	《石学敏针灸临证集验》	头痛（第156页）
35	石学敏	《当代针灸治疗学》	偏头痛（第102页）
36	卞金玲	《石学敏针灸学》	头痛（第374页）
37	田从豁	《针灸医学验集》	头痛（第454页）
38	田从豁	《中国灸法集粹》	头痛（第280页）
39	田从豁	《田从豁临床经验》	头痛（第60页）
40	刘志顺	《田从豁》	头痛（第45页）
41	王乐亭	《金针王乐亭》	头痛（第109页）
42	张俊英	《金针王乐亭经验集》	偏头痛（第45~46页）
43	王宏才	《针灸名家医案解读》	头痛（第34页）

5 文献质量评估结论

5.1 证据概要表(evidence profile,EP)

5.1.1 放血

放血 VS 西药

No of studies	Quality assessment						No of patients		Effect		Quality	Importance
	Design	Risk of bias	Inconsistency	Indirectness	Imprecision	Other considerations	Bleeding	Western medicine	Relative (95% CI)	Absolute		
HT－5 (Better indicated by lower values)												
1	randomised trials	serious[1,2]	no serious inconsistency	no serious indirectness	no serious imprecision	reporting bias[3]	50	40	-	MD 26.89 higher (21.77 to 32.01 higher)	⊕○○○ very low	important
NO (Better indicated by lower values)												
1	randomised trials	serious[1,2]	no serious inconsistency	no serious indirectness	no serious imprecision	reporting bias[3]	50	40	-	MD 34.83 lower (41.23 to 28.43 lower)	⊕○○○ very low	important
Degree of headache (Better indicated by lower values)												
1	randomised trials	serious[1,2]	no serious inconsistency	serious	no serious imprecision	reporting bias[3]	50	40	-	MD 0.9 lower (1.44 to 0.36 lower)	⊕○○○ very low	important
Lasting time (Better indicated by lower values)												
1	randomised trials	serious[1,2]	no serious inconsistency	serious	no serious imprecision	reporting bias[3]	50	40	-	MD 1.3 lower (1.67 to 0.93 lower)	⊕○○○ very low	important
Index of headache (Better indicated by lower values)												
1	randomised trials	serious[1,2]	serious	serious	no serious imprecision	reporting bias[3]	50	40	-	MD 1.8 lower (3.71 lower to 0.11 higher)	⊕○○○ very low	critical

Ineffective rate

No of studies	Quality assessment						No of patients		Effect		Quality	Importance
	Design	Risk of bias	Inconsistency	Indirectness	Imprecision	Other considerations	Bleeding	Western medicine	Relative (95% CI)	Absolute		
1	randomised trials	serious[1,2]	no serious inconsistency	serious	no serious imprecision	reporting bias[3]	3/50 (6%)	11/40 (27.5%)	OR 0.17 (0.04 to 0.65)	214 fewer per 1000 (from 77 fewer to 260 fewer)	⊕○○○ very low	important
							–	27.5%	(0.04 to 0.65)	214 fewer per 1000 (from 77 fewer to 260 fewer)		

1 there is no blinding method in both studies.
2 allocation consealment:one is good, the other is not so good.
3 the numbers of study are not enough.

放血 VS 常规针刺

Ineffective rate

No of studies	Quality assessment						No of patients		Effect		Quality	Importance
	Design	Risk of bias	Inconsistency	Indirectness	Imprecision	Other considerations	Bleeding	Common acupuncture	Relative (95% CI)	Absolute		
1	randomised trials	serious[1]	no serious inconsistency	no serious indirectness	serious	reporting bias[2]	2/54 (3.7%)	10/40 (25%)	OR 0.12 (0.02 to 0.56)	212 fewer per 1000 (from 93 fewer to 243 fewer)	⊕○○○ very low	important
							–	25%	(0.02 to 0.56)	212 fewer per 1000 (from 93 fewer to 243 fewer)		

VAS (Better indicated by lower values)

No of studies	Design	Risk of bias	Inconsistency	Indirectness	Imprecision	Other considerations	Bleeding	Common acupuncture	Relative (95% CI)	Absolute	Quality	Importance
1	randomised trials	serious[1,3]	no serious inconsistency	no serious indirectness	no serious imprecision	reporting bias[2]	54	40	–	MD 0.45 lower (0.91 lower to 0.01 higher)	⊕○○○ very low	critical

Frequency of attack (Better indicated by lower values)

No of studies	Design	Risk of bias	Inconsistency	Indirectness	Imprecision	Other considerations	Bleeding	Common acupuncture	Relative (95% CI)	Absolute	Quality	Importance
1	randomised trials	serious[1,3]	no serious inconsistency	serious	no serious imprecision	reporting bias[2]	54	40	–	MD 0.78 lower (1.27 to 0.29 lower)	⊕○○○ very low	important

Continued

Lasting time (Better indicated by lower values)

No of studies	Design	Risk of bias	Inconsistency	Indirectness	Imprecision	Other considerations	No of patients		Relative (95% CI)	Effect Absolute	Quality	Importance
1	randomised trials	serious[1,3]	no serious inconsistency	no serious indirectness	no serious imprecision	reporting bias[2]	54	40	–	MD 0.54 lower (1.02 to 0.06 lower)	⊕◯◯◯ very low	important

Symptoms (Better indicated by lower values)

No of studies	Design	Risk of bias	Inconsistency	Indirectness	Imprecision	Other considerations	No of patients		Relative (95% CI)	Effect Absolute	Quality	Importance
1	randomised trials	serious[1,3]	no serious inconsistency	no serious indirectness	no serious imprecision	reporting bias[2]	54	40	–	MD 0.51 lower (0.66 to 0.36 lower)	⊕◯◯◯ very low	important

1 allocation consealment:one is good, the other is not so good.

2 the numbers of study are not enough.

3 there is no blinding method in both studies.

耳穴放血 VS 西药 (发作期)

No of studies	Design	Quality assessment					No of patients		Effect		Quality	Importance
		Risk of bias	Inconsistency	Indirectness	Imprecision	Other considerations	Auricular point method	Western medicine	Relative (95% CI)	Absolute		

VAS (Better indicated by lower values)

1	randomised trials	serious[1,2]	no serious inconsistency	serious	no serious imprecision	reporting bias[3]	70	33	–	MD 8.03 higher (3.41 to 12.65 higher)	⊕◯◯◯ very low	critical

Relieving time (Better indicated by lower values)

1	randomised trials	serious[1,2]	no serious inconsistency	serious	no serious imprecision	reporting bias[3]	70	33	–	MD 15.29 lower (30.71 lower to 0.13 higher)	⊕◯◯◯ very low	important

1 there is no blinding method in both studies.

2 allocation consealment:one is good, the other is not so good.

3 the numbers of study are not enough.

耳穴放血 VS 西药（缓解期）

No of studies	Quality assessment						No of patients		Effect		Quality	Importance
	Design	Risk of bias	Inconsistency	Indirectness	Imprecision	Other considerations	Auricular point method	Western medicine	Relative	(95% CI) Absolute		
Score of headache (Better indicated by lower values)												
3	randomised trials	serious[1,2]	serious	no serious indirectness	no serious imprecision	reporting bias[3]	162	125	–	MD 4.15 higher (3.15 to 5.14 higher)	⊕○○○ very low	critical
Ineffective rate												
3	randomised trials	serious[1,2]	no serious inconsistency	no serious indirectness	serious	reporting bias[3]	17/162 (10.5%) / –	34/125 (27.2%) / 32.6%	OR 0.38 (0.2 to 0.72)	148 fewer per 1000 (from 60 fewer to 202 fewer) / 171 fewer per 1000 (from 68 fewer to 238 fewer)	⊕○○○ very low	important
HT – 5 (Better indicated by lower values)												
1	randomised trials	serious[1,2]	no serious inconsistency	serious	no serious imprecision	reporting bias[3]	46	46	–	MD 19.5 higher (12.72 to 26.28 higher)	⊕○○○ very low	important

1 there is no blinding method in both studies.

2 allocation consealment; one is good, the other is not so good.

3 the numbers of study are not enough.

5.1.2 毫针刺法（电针）
毫针刺 VS 西药（发作期）

No of studies	Design	Quality assessment					No of patients		Effect		Quality	Importance
		Risk of bias	Inconsistency	Indirectness	Imprecision	Other considerations	Acupuncture	Western medicine	Relative (95% CI)	Absolute		
VAS (Better indicated by lower values)												
1	randomised trials	serious[1,2]	no serious inconsistency	serious	no serious imprecision	reporting bias[3]	68	69	-	MD 1.14 higher (0.73 to 1.55 higher)	⊕◯◯◯ very low	critical
Ineffective rate												
1	randomised trials	serious[1]	no serious inconsistency	serious	serious	reporting bias[3]	3/68 (4.4%)	7/69 (10.1%)	OR 0.41 (0.1 to 1.65)	57 fewer per 1000 (from 90 fewer to 56 more)	⊕◯◯◯ very low	important
							-	10.1%		57 fewer per 1000 (from 90 fewer to 55 more)		
Number of patients avoid attack within 48h												
1	randomised trials	no serious risk of bias	no serious inconsistency	no serious indirectness	no serious imprecision	reporting bias[3]	21/60 (35%)	21/58 (36.2%)	OR 0.95 (0.45 to 2.02)	12 fewer per 1000 (from 159 fewer to 172 more)	⊕⊕⊕◯ moderate	critical
							-	36.2%		12 fewer per 1000 (from 159 fewer to 172 more)		
Adverse effect(n)												
1	randomised trials	no serious risk of bias	no serious inconsistency	no serious indirectness	no serious imprecision	reporting bias[3]	16/60 (26.7%)	36/58 (62.1%)	-	621 fewer per 1000 (from 621 fewer to 621 fewer)	⊕⊕⊕◯ moderate	important
							-	62.1%		621 fewer per 1000 (from 621 fewer to 621 fewer)		

1 there is no blinding method in both studies.

2 allocation consealment：one is good, the other is not so good.

3 the numbers of study are not enough.

毫针刺 VS 西药(缓解期)

No of studies	Quality assessment						No of patients		Effect		Quality	Importance
	Design	Risk of bias	Inconsistency	Indirectness	Imprecision	Other considerations	Acupuncture	Western medicine	Relative (95% CI)	Absolute		
Ineffective rate												
4	randomised trials	serious[1,2]	no serious inconsistency	no serious indirectness	no serious imprecision	reporting bias[3]	10/141 (7.1%)	38/139 (27.3%) / 27.6%	OR 0.2 (0.09 to 0.42)	203 fewer per 1000 (from 137 fewer to 241 fewer) / 205 fewer per 1000 (from 138 fewer to 243 fewer)	⊕⊕○○ low	important
Score of headache (Better indicated by lower values)												
2	randomised trials	serious[1,2]	serious	no serious indirectness	serious	reporting bias[4]	89	88	–	MD 3.2 lower (4.4 to 2 lower)	⊕○○○ very low	important
Lasting time (Better indicated by lower values)												
1	randomised trials	serious[1,2]	no serious inconsistency	no serious indirectness	serious	reporting bias[4]	32	31	–	MD 3.67 lower (5.04 to 2.3 lower)	⊕○○○ very low	important
Vas (Better indicated by lower values)												
1	randomised trials	serious[1,2]	no serious inconsistency	no serious indirectness	serious	reporting bias[4]	32	31	–	MD 0.53 lower (0.65 to 0.41 lower)	⊕○○○ very low	critical
Days of headache in one month (Follow-up 4~5 months; Better indicated by lower values)												
5	randomised trials	no serious risk of bias	serious[3,5]	no serious indirectness	serious[6]	reporting bias[4]	272	294	–	MD 1.26 lower (1.87 to 0.64 lower)	⊕○○○ very low	critical
Number of migraine attacks (Follow-up 2~4 months; Better indicated by lower values)												
2	randomised trials	no serious risk of bias	no serious inconsistency	no serious indirectness	no serious imprecision	reporting bias[4]	134	130	–	MD 1.13 lower (1.27 to 0.98 lower)	⊕⊕⊕○ moderate	critical

Continued

No of studies	Quality assessment						No of patients		Effect		Quality	Importance
	Design	Risk of bias	Inconsistency	Indirectness	Imprecision	Other considerations	Acupuncture	Western medicine	Relative (95% CI)	Absolute		

Physical status (Follow – up 2 ~ 3 months; measured with: SF – 36; Better indicated by higher values)

| 4 | randomised trials | no serious risk of bias | serious[3] | no serious indirectness | serious[3] | reporting bias[4] | 288 | 261 | – | MD 2.75 higher (1.47 to 7.02 higher) | ⊕◯◯◯ very low | important |

Side effect (Assessed with: number of patients)

| 4 | randomised trials | no serious risk of bias | serious[5] | no serious indirectness | no serious imprecision | reporting bias[4] | 26/239 (10.9%) | 94/227 (41.4%) | OR 0.16 (0.1 to 0.26) | 313 fewer per 1000 (from 259 fewer to 348 fewer) | ⊕⊕◯◯ low | important |
| | | | | | | | – | 41.4% | | 312 fewer per 1000 (from 259 fewer to 348 fewer) | | |

1 there is no blinding method in both studies.

2 allocation consealment;one is good, the other is not so good.

3 No explanation was provided.

4 the numbers of study are not enough.

5 the 95% CI of one study crosses with equivalent line but the other doesn't.

6 the ratio of effect size with 95% CI is between 50% ~ 90%.

毫针刺 VS 伪针刺（发作期）

No of studies	Quality assessment						No of patients		Effect		Quality	Importance
	Design	Risk of bias	Inconsistency	Indirectness	Imprecision	Other considerations	Acupuncture	Sham acupuncture	Relative (95% CI)	Absolute		
Intensity of headache (Measured with: VAS; Better indicated by lower values)												
2	randomised trials	no serious risk of bias	serious[1]	no serious indirectness	no serious imprecision	reporting bias[2,3]	131	132	–	MD 1.30 lower (1.99 to 0.62 lower)	⊕⊕◯◯ low	critical
Relief within 24 hours, n (%)												
1	randomised trials	no serious risk of bias	no serious inconsistency	no serious indirectness	very serious[4]	reporting bias[3]	22/54 (40.7%) / –	9/55 (16.4%) / 16.4%	OR 3.51 (1.43 to 8.62)	244 more per 1000 (from 55 more to 464 more) / 244 more per 1000 (from 55 more to 464 more)	⊕◯◯◯ very low	critical
Relapse or aggravation over 24 hours, n (%)												
1	randomised trials	no serious risk of bias	no serious inconsistency	no serious indirectness	serious[5]	reporting bias[3]	11/54 (20.4%) / –	29/55 (52.7%) / 52.70%	OR 0.23 (0.1 to 0.54)	323 fewer per 1000 (from 151 fewer to 427 fewer) / 323 fewer per 1000 (from 151 fewer to 427 fewer)	⊕⊕◯◯ low	critical
Headache score (24h after) (Measured with: McGill scale score; Better indicated by lower values)												
1	randomised trials	no serious risk of bias	no serious inconsistency	no serious indirectness	no serious imprecision	reporting bias[1]	75	75	–	MD 2.3 lower (3.52 to 1.08 lower)	⊕⊕⊕◯ moderate	critical
Medication (n)												
2	randomised trials	no serious risk of bias	serious[2]	no serious indirectness	no serious imprecision	reporting bias[3]	42/129 (32.6%) / –	77/130 (59.2%) / 59.2%	OR 0.31 (0.18 to 0.52)	282 fewer per 1000 (from 162 fewer to 385 fewer) / 282 fewer per 1000 (from 162 fewer to 385 fewer)	⊕⊕◯◯ low	critical

1 one study shows no significant different between two groups, while the other does.
2 No explanation was provided.
3 the number of study is not enough.
4 the ratio between effect size and 95% CI is lower than 50%.
5 the ratio between effect size and 95% CI is between 50% ~ 90%.

毫针刺 VS 伪针刺（缓解期）

No of studies	Quality assessment						No of patients		Effect		Quality	Importance
	Design	Risk of bias	Inconsistency	Indirectness	Imprecision	Other considerations	Acupuncture	Sham acupuncture	Relative (95% CI)	Absolute		
Headache days (Better indicated by lower values)												
3	randomised trials	no serious risk of bias	very serious[1]	no serious indirectness	serious[2]	reporting bias[3]	281	215	–	MD 0.61 lower (1.71 to 0.14 lower)	⊕◯◯◯ very low	critical
Number of headache attacks per month (Follow-up 1~3 months; Better indicated by lower values)												
2	randomised trials	no serious risk of bias	very serious[1]	no serious indirectness	very serious[4]	reporting bias[3]	171	168	–	MD 0.48 lower (0.7 to 0.27 lower)	⊕◯◯◯ very low	critical

1 effect sizes disseminate on both sides of the equivalent line.

2 the ratio of effect size and 95% CI is 50% ~ 90%.

3 the number of studies is not enough.

4 the ratio of effect size and 95% CI is <50%.

头针 VS 西药

No of studies	Quality assessment						No of patients		Effect		Quality	Importance
	Design	Risk of bias	Inconsistency	Indirectness	Imprecision	Other considerations	Scalp needle combined with western medicine	Western medicine	Relative (95% CI)	Absolute		
Ineffect rate												
1	randomised trials	serious[1,2]	no serious inconsistency	serious	no serious imprecision	reporting bias[3]	6/38 (15.8%)	28/42 (66.7%)	OR 0.09 (0.03 to 0.28)	514 fewer per 1000 (from 308 fewer to 610 fewer)	⊕◯◯◯ very low	important
							–	66.7%		514 fewer per 1000 (from 308 fewer to 610 fewer)		

VAS (Better indicated by lower values)

No of studies	Design	Risk of bias	Inconsistency	Indirectness	Imprecision	Other considerations	Fire needle	Electro-acupuncture	Relative (95% CI)	Absolute	Quality	Importance
1	randomised trials	serious[1,2]	no serious inconsistency	serious	no serious imprecision	reporting bias[3]	38	42	–	MD 2.58 higher (1.58 to 3.58 higher)	⊕◯◯◯ very low	critical

Score of TCM symptoms (Better indicated by lower values)

No of studies	Design	Risk of bias	Inconsistency	Indirectness	Imprecision	Other considerations	Fire needle	Electro-acupuncture	Relative (95% CI)	Absolute	Quality	Importance
1	randomised trials	serious[1,2]	no serious inconsistency	serious	no serious imprecision	reporting bias[3]	38	42	–	MD 2.74 higher (1.73 to 3.75 higher)	⊕◯◯◯ very low	important

1 there is no blinding method in both studies.
2 allocation consealment: one is good, the other is not so good.
3 the numbers of study are not enough.

5.1.3 火针
火针 VS 电针

No of studies	Design	Quality assessment					No of patients		Effect		Quality	Importance
		Risk of bias	Inconsistency	Indirectness	Imprecision	Other considerations	Fire needle	Electro-acupuncture	Relative (95% CI)	Absolute		

Ineffective rate

No of studies	Design	Risk of bias	Inconsistency	Indirectness	Imprecision	Other considerations	Fire needle	Electro-acupuncture	Relative (95% CI)	Absolute	Quality	Importance
1	randomised trials	serious[1,2]	no serious inconsistency	serious	no serious imprecision	reporting bias[3]	9/88 (10.2%)	12/44 (27.3%)	OR 0.3 (0.12 to 0.79)	172 fewer per 1000 (from 44 fewer to 230 fewer)	⊕◯◯◯ very low	important
							–	27.3%		172 fewer per 1000 (from 44 fewer to 230 fewer)		

1 there is no blinding method in both studies.
2 allocation consealment: one is good, the other is not so good.
3 the numbers of study are not enough.

5.2　结果总结表 (the summary of findings table, SoFs table)
5.2.1　放血
放血 VS 西药

Bleeding compared to western medicine for migraine

Patient or population: patients with migraine

Settings:

Intervention: bleeding

Comparison: western medicine

Outcomes	Illustrative comparative risks* (95% CI)		Relative effect (95% CI)	No of Participants (studies)	Quality of the evidence (GRADE)	Comments
	Assumed risk Western medicine	Corresponding risk Bleeding				
HT-5		The mean HT-5 in the intervention groups was 26.89 higher (21.77 to 32.01 higher)		90 (1 study)	⊕⊖⊖⊖ very low[1,2,3]	
NO		The mean NO in the intervention groups was 34.83 lower (41.23 to 28.43 lower)		90 (1 study)	⊕⊖⊖⊖ very low[1,2,3]	
Degree of headache		The mean degree of headache in the intervention groups was 0.9 lower (1.44 to 0.36 lower)		90 (1 study)	⊕⊖⊖⊖ very low[1,2,3]	
Lasting time		The mean lasting time in the intervention groups was 1.3 lower (1.67 to 0.93 lower)		90 (1 study)	⊕⊖⊖⊖ very low[1,2,3]	
Index of headache		The mean index of headache in the intervention groups was 1.8 lower (3.71 lower to 0.11 higher)		90 (1 study)	⊕⊖⊖⊖ very low[1,2,3]	

Continued

Ineffective rate				
Study population				
275 per 1000	61 per 1000 (15 to 198)	OR 0.17 (0.04 to 0.65)	90 (1 study)	⊕◯◯◯ very low[1,2,3]
Moderate				
275 per 1000	61 per 1000 (15 to 198)			

* The basis for the assumed risk (e. g. the median control group risk across studies) is provided in footnotes. The corresponding risk (and its 95% confidence interval) is based on the assumed risk in the comparison group and the relative effect of the intervention (and its 95% CI).

CI: Confidence interval; OR: Odds ratio.

GRADE Working Group grades of evidence

High quality: Further research is very unlikely to change our confidence in the estimate of effect.

Moderate quality: Further research is likely to have an important impact on our confidence in the estimate of effect and may change the estimate.

Low quality: Further research is very likely to have an important impact on our confidence in the estimate of effect and is likely to change the estimate.

Very low quality: We are very uncertain about the estimate.

1 there is no blinding method in both studies.

2 allocation consealment:one is good, the other is not so good.

3 the numbers of study are not enough.

放血 VS 常规针刺

Bleeding compared to common acupuncture for migraine

Patient or population: patients with migraine
Settings:
Intervention: bleeding
Comparison: common acupuncture

Outcomes	Illustrative comparative risks* (95% CI)		Relative effect (95% CI)	No of Participants (studies)	Quality of the evidence (GRADE)	Comments
	Assumed risk Common acupuncture	Corresponding risk Bleeding				
Ineffective rate	Study population		OR 0.12 (0.02 to 0.56)	94 (1 study)	⊕⊕⊝⊝ very low[1,2]	
	250 per 1000	38 per 1000 (7 to 157)				
	Moderate					
	250 per 1000	38 per 1000 (7 to 157)				
VAS	The mean VAS in the intervention groups was 0.45 lower (0.91 lower to 0.01 higher)			94 (1 study)	⊕⊕⊝⊝ very low[1,2,3]	
Frequency of attack	The mean frequency of attack in the intervention groups was 0.78 lower (1.27 to 0.29 lower)			94 (1 study)	⊕⊕⊝⊝ very low[1,2,3]	
Lasting time	The mean lasting time in the intervention groups was 0.54 lower (1.02 to 0.06 lower)			94 (1 study)	⊕⊕⊝⊝ very low[1,2,3]	
Symptoms	The mean symptoms in the intervention groups was 0.51 lower (0.66 to 0.36 lower)			94 (1 study)	⊕⊕⊝⊝ very low[1,2,3]	

Continued

* The basis for the assumed risk (e. g. the median control group risk across studies) is provided in footnotes. The corresponding risk (and its 95% confidence interval) is based on the assumed risk in the comparison group and the relative effect of the intervention (and its 95% CI).

CI: Confidence interval; OR: Odds ratio.

GRADE Working Group grades of evidence

High quality: Further research is very unlikely to change our confidence in the estimate of effect.

Moderate quality: Further research is likely to have an important impact on our confidence in the estimate of effect and may change the estimate.

Low quality: Further research is very likely to have an important impact on our confidence in the estimate of effect and is likely to change the estimate.

Very low quality: We are very uncertain about the estimate.

1 allocation consealment: one is good, the other is not so good.

2 the numbers of study are not enough.

3 there is no blinding method in both studies.

耳穴放血 VS 西药（发作期）

Auricular point method compared to western medicine for migraine

Patient or population: patients with migraine

Settings:

Intervention: auricular point method

Comparison: western medicine

Outcomes	Illustrative comparative risks* (95% CI)		Relative effect (95% CI)	No of Participants (studies)	Quality of the evidence (GRADE)	Comments
	Assumed risk	Corresponding risk				
	Western medicine	Auricular point method				
VAS		The mean VAS in the intervention groups was 8. 03 higher (3. 41 to 12. 65 higher)		103 (1 study)	⊕◯◯◯ very low[1,2,3]	
Relieving time		The mean relieving time in the intervention groups was 15. 29 lower (30. 71 lower to 0. 13 higher)		103 (1 study)	⊕◯◯◯ very low[1,2,3]	

* The basis for the assumed risk (e. g. the median control group risk across studies) is provided in footnotes. The corresponding risk (and its 95% confidence interval) is based on the assumed risk in the comparison group and the relative effect of the intervention (and its 95% CI).

CI: Confidence interval.

GRADE Working Group grades of evidence

High quality: Further research is very unlikely to change our confidence in the estimate of effect.

Moderate quality: Further research is likely to have an important impact on our confidence in the estimate of effect and may change the estimate.

Low quality: Further research is very likely to have an important impact on our confidence in the estimate of effect and is likely to change the estimate.

Very low quality: We are very uncertain about the estimate.

1 there is no blinding method in both studies.

2 allocation consealment: one is good, the other is not so good.

3 the numbers of study are not enough.

耳穴放血 VS 西药（缓解期）

Auricular point method compared to western medicine for migraine

Patient or population: patients with migraine

Settings:

Intervention: auricular point method

Comparison: western medicine

Outcomes	Illustrative comparative risks * (95% CI)		Relative effect (95% CI)	No of Participants (studies)	Quality of the evidence (GRADE)	Comments
	Assumed risk	Corresponding risk				
	Western medicine	Auricular point method				
Score of headache		The mean score of headache in the intervention groups was 4.15 higher (3.15 to 5.14 higher)		287 (3 studies)	⊕⊖⊖⊖ very low[1,2,3]	
Ineffective rate	Study population		OR 0.38 (0.2 to 0.72)	287 (3 studies)	⊕⊖⊖⊖ very low[1,2,3]	
	272 per 1000	124 per 1000 (70 to 212)				
	Moderate					
	326 per 1000	155 per 1000 (88 to 258)				
HT – 5		The mean HT – 5 in the intervention groups was 19.5 higher (12.72 to 26.28 higher)		92 (1 study)	⊕⊖⊖⊖ very low[1,2,3]	

* The basis for the assumed risk (e. g. the median control group risk across studies) is provided in footnotes. The corresponding risk (and its 95% confidence interval) is based on the assumed risk in the comparison group and the relative effect of the intervention (and its 95% CI).

CI: Confidence interval; OR: Odds ratio.

GRADE Working Group grades of evidence

High quality: Further research is very unlikely to change our confidence in the estimate of effect.

Moderate quality: Further research is likely to have an important impact on our confidence in the estimate of effect and may change the estimate.

Low quality: Further research is very likely to have an important impact on our confidence in the estimate of effect and is likely to change the estimate.

Very low quality: We are very uncertain about the estimate.

1 there is no blinding method in both studies.

2 allocation consealment；one is good, the other is not so good.

3 the numbers of study are not enough.

5.2.2 毫针刺法（电针）
毫针刺 VS 西药（发作期）

Acupuncture compared to western medicine for migraine

Patient or population: patients with migraine
Settings:
Intervention: acupuncture
Comparison: western medicine

Outcomes	Illustrative comparative risks* (95% CI)		Relative effect (95% CI)	No of Participants (studies)	Quality of the evidence (GRADE)	Comments
	Assumed risk Western medicine	Corresponding risk Acupuncture				
VAS		The mean VAS in the intervention groups was 1.14 higher (0.73 to 1.55 higher)		137 (1 study)	⊕⊕⊝⊝ very low[1,2,3]	
Ineffective rate	Study population		OR 0.41 (0.1 to 1.65)	137 (1 study)	⊕⊕⊝⊝ very low[1,3]	
	101 per 1000	44 per 1000 (11 to 157)				
	Moderate					
	101 per 1000	44 per 1000 (11 to 156)				
Number of patients avoid attack within 48h	Study population		OR 0.95 (0.45 to 2.02)	118 (1 study)	⊕⊕⊕⊝ moderate[3]	
	362 per 1000	350 per 1000 (203 to 534)				
	Moderate					
	362 per 1000	350 per 1000 (203 to 534)				
Adverse effect(n)	Study population		Not estimable	118 (1 study)	⊕⊕⊕⊝ moderate[3]	
	621 per 1000	0 per 1000 (0 to 0)				
	Moderate					
	621 per 1000	0 per 1000 (0 to 0)				

Continued

* The basis for the assumed risk (e. g. the median control group risk across studies) is provided in footnotes. The corresponding risk (and its 95% confidence interval) is based on the assumed risk in the comparison group and the relative effect of the intervention (and its 95% CI).

CI: Confidence interval; RR: Risk ratio; OR: Odds ratio.

GRADE Working Group grades of evidence

High quality: Further research is very unlikely to change our confidence in the estimate of effect.

Moderate quality: Further research is likely to have an important impact on our confidence in the estimate of effect and may change the estimate.

Low quality: Further research is very likely to have an important impact on our confidence in the estimate of effect and is likely to change the estimate.

Very low quality: We are very uncertain about the estimate.

1 there is no blinding method in both studies.

2 allocation consealment:one is good, the other is not so good.

3 the numbers of study are not enough.

毫针刺 VS 西药（缓解期）

Acupuncture compared to western medicine for migraine

Patient or population: patients with migraine
Settings:
Intervention: acupuncture
Comparison: western medicine

Outcomes	Illustrative comparative risks * (95% CI)		Relative effect (95% CI)	No of Participants (studies)	Quality of the evidence (GRADE)	Comments
	Assumed risk	Corresponding risk				
	Western medicine	Acupuncture				
Ineffective rate	Study population		OR 0.2 (0.09 to 0.42)	280 (4 studies)	⊕⊕⊕⊝ low[1,2,3]	
	273 per 1000	70 per 1000 (33 to 136)				
	Moderate					
	276 per 1000	71 per 1000 (33 to 138)				
Score of headache		The mean score of headache in the intervention groups was 3.2 lower (4.4 to 2 lower)		177 (2 studies)	⊕⊝⊝⊝ very low[1,2,4]	
Lasting time		The mean lasting time in the intervention groups was 3.67 lower (5.04 to 2.3 lower)		63 (1 study)	⊕⊝⊝⊝ very low[1,2,4]	
VAS		The mean VAS in the intervention groups was 0.53 lower (0.65 to 0.41 lower)		63 (1 study)	⊕⊕⊕⊝ very low[1,2,4]	
Days of headache in one month Follow-up: 4~5 months	The mean days of headache in one month ranged across control groups from -1.5 ~ -7.9 day.	The mean days of headache in one month in the intervention groups was 1.26 lower (1.87 to 0.64 lower)		566 (5 studies)	⊕⊝⊝⊝ very low[3,4,5,6]	

Continued

	Assumed risk (Control)	Corresponding risk (Intervention)	Relative effect (95% CI)	No of Participants (studies)	Quality of evidence (GRADE)
Number of migraine attacks Follow – up: 2 ~ 4 months	The mean number of migraine attacks ranged across control groups from 2.4 ~ 4.1 time	The mean number of migraine attacks in the intervention groups was 1.13 lower (1.27 to 0.98 lower)		264 (2 studies)	⊕⊕⊕⊝ moderate[4]
Physical status SF – 36 Follow – up: 2 ~ 3 months	The mean physical status ranged across control groups from 44.5 ~ 54.8 score	The mean physical status in the intervention groups was 2.75 higher (1.47 to 7.02 higher)		549 (4 studies)	⊕⊕⊝⊝ very low[3,4]
Side effect Number of patients	Study population 414 per 1000	102 per 1000 (66 to 155)	OR 0.16 (0.1 to 0.26)	466 (4 studies)	⊕⊕⊝⊝ low[4,5]
	Moderate 414 per 1000	102 per 1000 (66 to 155)			

* The basis for the assumed risk (e.g. the median control group risk across studies) is provided in footnotes. The corresponding risk (and its 95% confidence interval) is based on the assumed risk in the comparison group and the relative effect of the intervention (and its 95% CI).

CI: Confidence interval; OR: Odds ratio.

GRADE Working Group grades of evidence

High quality: Further research is very unlikely to change our confidence in the estimate of effect.

Moderate quality: Further research is likely to have an important impact on our confidence in the estimate of effect and may change the estimate.

Low quality: Further research is very likely to have an important impact on our confidence in the estimate of effect and is likely to change the estimate.

Very low quality: We are very uncertain about the estimate.

1 there is no blinding method in both studies.

2 allocation consealment: one is good, the other is not so good.

3 No explanation was provided.

4 the numbers of study are not enough.

5 the 95% CI of one study crosses with equivalent line but the other doesn't.

6 the ratio of effect size with 95% CI is between 50% ~ 90%.

毫针刺 VS 伪针刺(发作期)

Acupuncture compared to sham acupuncture for migraine

Patient or population: migraine
Settings:
Intervention: acupuncture
Comparison: sham acupuncture

Outcomes	Illustrative comparative risks* (95% CI)		Relative effect (95% CI)	No of Participants (studies)	Quality of the evidence (GRADE)	Comments
	Assumed risk	Corresponding risk				
	Sham acupuncture	Acupuncture				
Intensity of headache VAS	The mean intensity of headache in the control groups was 4.9 score	The mean intensity of headache in the intervention groups was 1.30 lower (1.99 to 0.62 lower)		263 (2 studies)	⊕⊕⊕⊝ low[1,2,3]	
Relief within 24 hours, n (%)	Study population		OR 3.51 (1.43 to 8.62)	109 (1 study)	⊕⊝⊝⊝ very low[3,4]	
	164 per 1000	407 per 1000 (219 to 628)				
	Moderate					
	164 per 1000	408 per 1000 (219 to 628)				
Relapse or aggravation over 24 hours, n (%)	Study population		OR 0.23 (0.1 to 0.54)	109 (1 study)	⊕⊕⊝⊝ low[3,5]	
	527 per 1000	204 per 1000 (100 to 376)				
	Moderate					
	527 per 1000	204 per 1000 (100 to 376)				
Headache score(24h after) McGill scale score	The mean headache score(24h after) in the control groups was 6.4 score	The mean headache score(24h after) in the intervention groups was 2.3 lower (3.52 to 1.08 lower)		150 (1 study)	⊕⊕⊕⊝ moderate[1]	

Continued

Medication(n)	Study population			
	592 per 1000	311 per 1000 (207 to 430)		
	Moderate		OR 0.31 (0.18 to 0.52)	259 (2 studies)
	592 per 1000	310 per 1000 (207 to 430)		⊕⊕⊝⊝ low[2,3]

* The basis for the assumed risk (e. g. the median control group risk across studies) is provided in footnotes. The corresponding risk (and its 95% confidence interval) is based on the assumed risk in the comparison group and the relative effect of the intervention (and its 95% CI).
CI: Confidence interval; OR: Odds ratio.

GRADE Working Group grades of evidence
High quality: Further research is very unlikely to change our confidence in the estimate of effect.
Moderate quality: Further research is likely to have an important impact on our confidence in the estimate of effect and may change the estimate.
Low quality: Further research is very likely to have an important impact on our confidence in the estimate of effect and is likely to change the estimate.
Very low quality: We are very uncertain about the estimate.

1 one study shows no significant different between two groups, while the other does.
2 No explanation was provided.
3 the number of study is not enough.
4 the ratio between effect size and 95% CI is lower than 50%.
5 the ratio between effect size and 95% CI is between 50% ~90%.

毫针刺 VS 伪针刺（缓解期）

Acupuncture compared to sham acupuncture for

Patient or population:
Settings:
Intervention: acupuncture
Comparison: sham acupuncture

Outcomes	Illustrative comparative risks* (95% CI)		Relative effect (95% CI)	No of Participants (studies)	Quality of the evidence (GRADE)	Comments
	Assumed risk	Corresponding risk				
	Sham acupuncture	Acupuncture				
Headache days	The mean headache days ranged across control groups from 3.4 ~ 4.7 day	The mean headache days in the intervention groups was 0.61 lower (1.71 to 0.14 lower)		496 (3 studies)	⊕⊕⊝⊝ very low[1,2,3]	
Number of headacheattacks per month Follow – up: 1 ~ 3 months	The mean number of headacheattacks per month ranged across control groups from 1.7 ~ 4.6 time	The mean number of headacheattacks per month in the intervention groups was 0.48 lower (0.7 to 0.27 lower)		339 (2 studies)	⊕⊕⊝⊝ very low[1,3,4]	

* The basis for the assumed risk (e.g. the median control group risk across studies) is provided in footnotes. The corresponding risk (and its 95% confidence interval) is based on the assumed risk in the comparison group and the relative effect of the intervention (and its 95% CI).
CI: Confidence interval.

GRADE Working Group grades of evidence
High quality: Further research is very unlikely to change our confidence in the estimate of effect.
Moderate quality: Further research is likely to have an important impact on our confidence in the estimate of effect and may change the estimate.
Low quality: Further research is very likely to have an important impact on our confidence in the estimate of effect and is likely to change the estimate.
Very low quality: We are very uncertain about the estimate.

1 effect sizes disseminate on both sides of the equivalent line.
2 the ratio of effect size and 95% CI is 50% ~90%.
3 the number of studies is not enough.
4 the ratio of effect size and 95% CI is <50%.

头针 VS 西药

Scalp needle combined with western medicine compared to western medicine for migraine

Patient or population: patients with migraine
Settings:
Intervention: scalp needle combined with western medicine
Comparison: western medicine

Outcomes	Illustrative comparative risks* (95% CI)		Relative effect (95% CI)	No of Participants (studies)	Quality of the evidence (GRADE)	Comments
	Assumed risk	Corresponding risk				
	Western medicine	Scalp needle combined with western medicine				
Ineffect rate	Study population					
	667 per 1000	153 per 1000 (57 to 359)	OR 0.09 (0.03 to 0.28)	80 (1 study)	⊕⊝⊝⊝ very low[1,2,3]	
	Moderate					
	667 per 1000	153 per 1000 (57 to 359)				
VAS		The mean vas in the intervention groups was 2.58 higher (1.58 to 3.58 higher)		80 (1 study)	⊕⊝⊝⊝ very low[1,2,3]	
Score of TCM symptoms		The mean score of tcm symptoms in the intervention groups was 2.74 higher (1.73 to 3.75 higher)		80 (1 study)	⊕⊝⊝⊝ very low[1,2,3]	

* The basis for the assumed risk (e. g. the median control group risk across studies) is provided in footnotes. The corresponding risk (and its 95% confidence interval) is based on the assumed risk in the comparison group and the relative effect of the intervention (and its 95% CI).

CI: Confidence interval; OR: Odds ratio.

GRADE Working Group grades of evidence
High quality: Further research is very unlikely to change our confidence in the estimate of effect.
Moderate quality: Further research is likely to have an important impact on our confidence in the estimate of effect and may change the estimate.
Low quality: Further research is very likely to have an important impact on our confidence in the estimate of effect and is likely to change the estimate.
Very low quality: We are very uncertain about the estimate.

1 there is no blinding method in both studies.
2 allocation consealment; one is good, the other is not so good.
3 the numbers of study are not enough.

5.2.3 火针

火针 VS 电针

Fire needle compared to electro – acupuncture for migraine

Patient or population: patients with migraine

Settings:

Intervention: fire needle

Comparison: electro – acupuncture

Outcomes	Illustrative comparative risks * (95% CI)		Relative effect (95% CI)	No of Participants (studies)	Quality of the evidence (GRADE)	Comments
	Assumed risk	Corresponding risk				
	Electro – acupuncture	Fire needle				
Ineffective rate	Study population		OR 0.3 (0. 12 to 0. 79)	132 (1 study)	⊕⊖⊖⊖ very low[1,2,3]	
	273 per 1000	101 per 1000 (43 to 229)				
	Moderate					
	273 per 1000	101 per 1000 (43 to 229)				

* The basis for the assumed risk (e. g. the median control group risk across studies) is provided in footnotes. The corresponding risk (and its 95% confidence interval) is based on the assumed risk in the comparison group and the relative effect of the intervention (and its 95% CI).

CI: Confidence interval; OR: Odds ratio.

GRADE Working Group grades of evidence

High quality: Further research is very unlikely to change our confidence in the estimate of effect.

Moderate quality: Further research is likely to have an important impact on our confidence in the estimate of effect and may change the estimate.

Low quality: Further research is very likely to have an important impact on our confidence in the estimate of effect and is likely to change the estimate.

Very low quality: We are very uncertain about the estimate.

1 there is no blinding method in both studies.

2 allocation consealment; one is good, the other is not so good.

3 the numbers of study are not enough.

6 本《指南》推荐方案的形成过程

由项目组组长和专家组成员根据《指南》的适用范围和临床问题确定《指南》推荐方案的框架。基本的框架在确定的基础上，按照偏头痛病程分期进行分类。在此基础上，按照干预措施再次分类。

证据的合成根据疾病的特点，按照不同目标人群、疾病的不同阶段、不同的治疗原则与针灸方法、疗效评价指标等因素，将现代文献根据 GRADE 系统评价形成治疗方案的推荐强度和推荐意见，结合古代文献及名医家经验证据进行归类，对于临床应用广泛，疗效明显但缺乏现代文献证据的治疗方法，在名医家经验和古代文献的基础上，通过专家共识的方法，形成推荐意见。再合并形成证据群。

推荐方案包括针灸干预的适用人群、介入时机、干预原则、取穴、针灸方法、注意事项、疗效及其评价指标等。每一条推荐意见都应有相对应的推荐强度和支撑证据。推荐意见的强度可分为强推荐、弱推荐两个层次。推荐意见的支撑证据包括现代文献证据、古代文献证据、名医家经验和专家共识。在每一条推荐方案的最后有相应的解释方案推荐的过程。

每一条推荐意见都从以下几个方面考虑：现代文献证据质量分级、古代文献证据及名医家经验可靠程度、干预措施的利弊关系、患者价值观和意愿、费用。

由项目组召开专家会议，逐条对针灸治疗疾病的介入时机、适用人群、治疗原则、各种针灸方法及其疗效及安全性等进行讨论，采用德尔菲法进行表决，筛选推荐方案，产生推荐意见。

7 本《指南》推荐方案征求意见稿

7.1 2008 版偏头痛针灸实践指南专家意见征集稿

下表是针灸治疗偏头痛的选穴和疗法处方，请您逐项进行评估。在"认可""可有可无"或"不认可"栏内以"√"来进行选择。在意见栏内表示您对该项具体的意见和建议。

治疗篇	认可	可有可无	不认可	意见
常规针刺方法 1：电针 取穴：太阳（双侧） 疗程：留针 30 分钟，每日 1 次，5 日为 1 个疗程，共治疗 4 个疗程，疗程间隔 2 日				
常规针刺方法 2：电针 取穴：双侧合谷、太冲 疗程：留针 30 分钟，3 次/周，治疗 4 周 本法适用于：无先兆偏头痛				
常规针刺方法 3：毫针刺 取穴：调神法（内关、人中、神门、百会）、丝竹空透率谷、太阳、风池、合谷、太冲、足临泣 疗程：留针 30 分钟，发作期每日 1 次，缓解期隔日 1 次，10 次为 1 个疗程				
常规针刺方法 4：毫针刺 取穴：对侧顶颞后斜线下 2/5、双侧顶旁 2 线。额颞部痛配同侧率谷、后枕，头顶痛配同侧风池 疗程：留针 30 分钟～1 小时，每日 1 次，10 次为 1 个疗程 本法适用于：无先兆偏头痛				

治疗篇	认可	可有可无	不认可	意见
特殊针刺方法 1：透刺法 主穴：丝竹空透率谷 配穴：太冲、足临泣、外关、丰隆、头维、风池、角孙 疗程：留针 20 分钟，每日 1 次，2 周为 1 个疗程 本法适用于：发作期偏头痛				
特殊针刺方法 2：透刺法 主穴：丝竹空透率谷、颔厌透悬颅 配穴：风池、列缺、太阳。水不涵木型加太溪、太冲；痰热内阻型加丰隆、外关；肝风上扰型加行间、合谷 疗程：留针 30 分钟，每日 1 次，10 次 1 个疗程，休息 5 天后再行第 2 疗程，共 3 个疗程 本法适用于：无先兆偏头痛				
特殊针刺方法 3：透刺法 取穴：太阳透率谷、头临泣透正营、上星透百会、脑空透风池、合谷透后溪 疗程：留针 30 分钟，每日 1 次，15 次为 1 个疗程 本法适用于：发作期中、重度偏头痛（瘀阻脑络证）				
特殊针刺方法 4：苍龟探穴法 采用局部取穴与远端循经取穴相结合 主穴：率谷、丝竹空、太阳、角孙 配穴：阳陵泉、太冲、足临泣、外关 疗程：留针 30 分钟，发作期每日 1 次，缓解期每 3 日 1 次 本法适用于：发作期偏头痛				
特殊针刺方法 5：贺氏三通法 微通法取穴：丝竹空透率谷、合谷、列缺、足临泣、风池、中脘、悬钟 温通法取穴：阿是穴、气海 强通法取穴：头维、太阳、攒竹 疗程：6 天为 1 个疗程，休息 1 天后进行下一疗程，共治疗 3 个疗程 本法适用于：无先兆偏头痛和有先兆偏头痛				

治疗篇	认可	可有可无	不认可	意见
其他针灸方法1：穴位注射结合刺络拔罐 穴位注射：丝竹空透率谷、风池 刺络拔罐：太阳穴处显露的浅静脉、阿是穴（患处压痛点、敏感点、结节或显露的浅静脉） 穴位注射药物：川芎嗪注射液 疗程：以上两法交替使用，每日1次，7天为1个疗程。疗程间休息1天，共4个疗程				
其他针灸方法2：火针结合电针 取穴：患侧头维、率谷、阿是穴，双侧阳池、丘墟 疗程：3日1次，3次为1个疗程，疗程间休息10天				
其他针灸方法3：耳穴综合疗法 耳背放血：耳背上1/3区血管充盈搏动处 自血穴注：风池、阳陵泉 耳穴点刺：标准耳穴的定位的颞（枕）、胰胆、神门、交感、皮质下、内分泌穴 本法适用于：发作期普通偏头痛的即刻止痛				
不同严重程度偏头痛的针灸疗效比较意见1：头痛程度越重，疗效越好				
不同严重程度偏头痛的针灸疗效比较意见2：头痛程度越轻，疗效越好				

7.2　2014版偏头痛针灸临床实践指南专家意见问卷

尊敬的专家：

您好！感谢您抽出宝贵的时间阅读并回答本问卷。本问卷（共三部分）需要征集您的意见：①治疗原则；②治疗方案；③方案排序。

推荐方案来源：基于针灸临床治疗偏头痛的中英文现代文献、古代文献、近现代名老中医经验，以及《指南》编写小组内的专家意见共识。

证据质量产生：本《指南》中英文现代文献采用 GRADE 系统为证据评级以衡量证据质量。GRADE 为《指南》提供了一个证据质量评价的体系，也为《指南》中的推荐强度评级提供了一种系统方法。GRADE 通过定性分析证据的偏移风险，并通过 META 分析进行定量评估，将证据质量分为高、中、低、极低四个等级，分别用 A、B、C、D 表示。证据质量 A：未来研究几乎不可能改变现有疗效评价结果的可信度；证据质量 B：未来研究可能对现有疗效评估有重要影响，可能改变评价结果的可信度；证据质量 C：表示未来研究很有可能对现有疗效评价有重要影响，改变评估结果可信度的可能性较大；证据质量 D：表示任何疗效评估都很不确定。

推荐强度根据：《指南》推荐需考虑到四方面因素，即证据质量、利弊平衡、患者意愿价值观、资源消耗与成本分析。请您根据四方面综合考虑后最终给出推荐强度。注：现有推荐方案仅对其证据质量进行了客观评级。GRADE 推荐强度建议采用数字1、2描述法：支持使用某项干预措施的强推荐1；支持使用某项干预措施的弱推荐2；反对使用某项干预措施的弱推荐2；反对使用某项干预措施的强推荐1。

注:

GRADE 为系统评价和《指南》提供了一个证据质量评价的体系，同时为《指南》中的推荐强度评级提供了一种系统方法。GRADE 在对文献中的各种临床结局指标分类基础上进行证据分级评估。在《指南》制定中，将证据分级综合其他方面因素，并最终形成推荐意见。GRADE 判断证据质量不是针对单个研究而是针对证据群。

GRADE 的证据质量判断根据：

证据群的偏倚风险：包括随机分组、隐蔽分组、盲法、结果数据的完整性、利益相关性等。

其他有关因素：包括证据质量的精确性、证据之间临床结果的一致性、临床结果的间接性及是否存在发表偏倚。

与观察性研究有关的另一些因素，包括效应量大小与量效关系的存在与否。

注：了解更多 GRADE 相关信息，请参考 http：//www. gradeworkinggroup. org。

META 分析

将同一临床问题的单个研究进行综合的统计学分析，目的是为了将结果进行合并，是一种合并几个试验结果的统计学方法。

偏头痛发作期及缓解期治疗方案

请您对于针灸治疗偏头痛的总治疗原则,治疗方法(取穴,操作,疗程)分别进行推荐,如果同意请选择"是(√)",如不同意请选择"否(√)"并同时填写否定理由或建议。并于最后对采用疗法进行排序推荐。请在表中"( )"内画"√"选择。

第一部分:治疗原则

1. 基于中英文现代文献证据支持

GRADE 证据评级基于 2 项 Meta 分析(纳入 5 个随机对照研究 RCT)

GRADE 评级为 C D

2. 有相关的名老中医经验支持及古代文献支持

		是否同意	不同意请写明原因或提供建议
治疗原则	调和气血,通络止痛。发作期以行气活血,通络止痛为主。缓解期以调和气血,疏通少阳为主	是( )否( )	理由: 建议:
选穴处方原则	急性期以少阳经、颞部及眼周局部阿是穴为主,配合远端取穴及耳穴。缓解期辨经配穴	是( )否( )	理由: 建议:
针刺干预时机	发作期和缓解期	是( )否( )	理由: 建议:

第二部分:治疗方案

发作期

一、针刺(电针)

1. 基于中英文现代文献证据支持

GRADE 证据评级基于 5 项 Meta 分析(纳入 5 个随机对照研究 RCT)

针刺优于西药:①降低 VAS;②改善无效率

常规针刺优于伪针刺:降低 VAS

GRADE 评级为 C D

2. 本疗法有相关的古代文献支持

治疗方案	方案一:阿是穴强刺激		
		是否同意	不同意请写明原因或提供建议
穴位:阿是穴		是( )否( )	否定理由:

操作:①定穴:选1~2个阿是穴。若疼痛是从一点逐渐散向周围,此点即为针刺部位;若疼痛区中心位置为针刺部位;若疼痛面积较大,无法定位,则通过寻痛找到压痛点明显或头皮肿胀点,以此为针刺部位。②手法:患者取坐位或卧位均可。常规消毒进针,选用直径0.30mm、长40mm毫针,对准穴位,与头皮呈30°角快速进针;进针后边以200r/min均匀快速向右捻转,并嘱患者根据针下感觉自行调节呼吸,即行针至此点时,患者瞬间使针尖在原位,摇拉上下小幅度提插1分钟;得气后将针稍提,用拇食指夹持针柄,再重上述不断震颤使针身弯曲成弩弓之状,针尖停留在得气点直至得气感消减弱,中指侧适当地弹击针体,摇拉行气,反复行针1分钟,留针时间1小时,使针感区域尽可能扩大,留针期间需要按照操作方法行针1~2次	是( )否( )	否定理由: 1. 定穴: 2. 手法: 3. 留针时间: 4. 其他原因及建议:
推荐意见:发作期偏头痛即刻止痛建议使用阿是穴强刺激	是( )否( )	否定理由:
方案二:透穴针刺		
取穴:太阳透率谷,头临泣透正营,上星透百会,脑空透风池,合谷透后溪。头部取穴以患侧为主,远端穴位双侧取穴	是( )否( )	否定理由: 1. 应去掉穴位: 2. 应增加穴位: 3. 其他原因及建议:
操作:①手法:患者取坐位或仰卧位。太阳透率谷,由太阳进针,平刺透向率谷;头临泣透正营,由头临泣进针,平刺透向正营;上星透百会,由上星进针,平刺透向百会;脑空透风池,由脑空进针,平刺透向风池;合谷透后溪,由合谷进针,直刺透后溪。以上透刺均进1.5~2寸,行小幅度快频率捻转,各行针1分钟。每次留针30分钟。留针期间需要按照操作方法行针1~2次②结合电针疗法,可提高疗效(专家共识)	是( )否( )	否定理由: 1. 患者体位: 2. 留针时间: 3. 手法: 4. 其他原因及建议:
推荐意见:发作期偏头痛中、重度偏头痛推荐使用透穴针刺结合电针治疗	是( )否( )	否定理由:
是否推荐针刺(电针)治疗 1. 强推荐( ) 2. 弱推荐( ) 3. 强不推荐( ) 4. 弱不推荐( ) 如果选择3. 强不推荐或4. 弱不推荐,请您说明理由:		

二、放血

1. 基于中英文现代文献证据支持

GRADE 证据评级基于 4 项 Meta 分析(纳入 6 个随机对照研究 RCT)

放血治疗优于西药:①降低 VAS;②加快疼痛缓解时间;③降低无效率;④降低头痛指数;⑤提高 5-HT、NO 含量

放血治疗优于常规针法:①降低 VAS;②降低无效率;③降低发作频率

GRADE 评级为 D

2. 本疗法有相关的古代文献和名老中医经验支持

治疗方案	是否同意	不同意请写明原因或提供建议
方案一:局部刺络		
穴位:局部压痛点或太阳穴周围浅表络脉	是( )否( )	否定理由: 1. 应去掉穴位: 2. 应增加穴位: 3. 其他原因及建议:
操作:①针具:三棱针;②手法:局部皮肤常规消毒后,左手拇、食指固定穴位周围皮肤,右手持三棱针点刺出血,挤出血时同时用75%酒精棉球擦拭局部,出血数滴后消毒脱脂棉按压止血	是( )否( )	否定理由: 1. 针具: 2. 手法: 3. 其他原因及建议:
推荐意见:发作期偏头痛可使用局部刺络法,并可配合常规针刺。缓解期也可参照治疗	是( )否( )	否定理由:
方案二:耳郭刺血		
取穴:耳背上 1/3 血管充盈处及颞(枕)、腆胆、神门、交感、皮质下、内分泌穴	是( )否( )	否定理由: 1. 应去掉穴位: 2. 应增加穴位: 3. 其他原因及建议:
操作:①针具:三棱针;②操作:耳背上 1/3 血管充盈处;先在耳背处按摩 3~5 分钟,使耳背明显充血,医者用左手拇指和中指固定耳郭,在耳背上 1/3 区以右手示指指腹触及血络,血管无充盈处,用指甲在所选部位掐印标记定位,局部常规消毒后用三棱针点刺出血,出血数滴。使之呈轻微点状出血,三棱针点刺后,局部常规消毒后用消毒脱脂棉按压	是( )否( )	否定理由: 1. 药物处理: 2. 其他原因及建议:
推荐意见:发作期偏头痛刻止痛建议使用耳郭刺血法	是( )否( )	否定理由:

是否推荐放血治疗
1. 强推荐（）2. 弱推荐（）3. 强不推荐（）4. 弱不推荐（）
如果选择3. 强不推荐或4. 弱不推荐，请您说明理由：

三、火针

1. 基于中英文现代文献证据支持
GRADE 证据评级基于 1 项 Meta 分析（纳入 1 个随机对照研究）
火针治疗优于电针：降低治疗无效率
GRADE 评级为 D
2. 本疗法有相关的名老中医经验支持

治疗方案	是否同意	不同意请写明原因或提供建议
取穴 阿是穴，头维（患侧），率谷（患侧）	是（）否（）	否定理由： 1. 应去掉穴位： 2. 应增加穴位： 3. 其他原因及建议：
操作：①针具：采用中号火针；②手法：穴位常规消毒，将针身的前中段烧至通红，对准阿是穴、患侧头维及率谷穴迅速刺入0.2～0.3寸并拔出，出针后用消毒干棉球按压针孔片刻	是（）否（）	否定理由： 1. 针具： 2. 手法： 3. 其他原因及建议：
推荐建议：发作期偏头痛可使用火针疗法，并可配合常规针刺。缓解期也可参考使用	是（）否（）	否定理由：

是否推荐火针治疗
1. 强推荐（）2. 弱推荐（）3. 强不推荐（）4. 弱不推荐（）
如果选择3. 强不推荐或4. 弱不推荐，请您说明理由：

缓解期

基于中英文现代文献证据支持
GRADE 证据评级基于 15 项 Meta 分析（纳入 13 个随机对照研究 RCT）
针灸优于西药：①降低无效率；②缩短头痛持续时间
头针加西药优于西药：①降低无效率；②缩短头痛持续时间；③降低头痛积分
GRADE 评级为 C D
本疗法有相关古代文献、名老中医经验支持

针灸综合治疗	是否同意	不同意请写明原因或提供建议

续表

取穴:穴方一 主穴:丝竹空、攒竹、太阳、风池、合谷、太冲、足临泣 配穴:阳陵泉、外关	是( )否( )	否定理由: 1. 应去掉穴位: 2. 应增加穴位: 3. 其他原因及建议:
穴方二 主穴:对侧顶颞后斜线下2/5,双侧顶旁2线 配穴:额部痛配同侧率谷,头项痛配同侧风池	是( )否( )	否定理由: 1. 应去掉穴位: 2. 应增加穴位: 3. 其他原因及建议::
在上述二方基础上,兼有厥阴经症状者:加内关、人中、神门,百会;兼有阳明经症状者:加头维;肝阳上亢型:加颔厌透悬颅,列缺,太溪,行间,内关;瘀血型:加颔厌透悬颅,头临泣;气血不足型:加足三里,气海,三阴交,太溪,肾俞;血海、足三里、三阴交;肾俞、膈俞,局部取穴中,远端取穴位。上述穴位中,局部取穴。	是( )否( )	否定理由: 1. 应去掉穴位: 2. 应增加穴位: 3. 其他原因及建议:
操作:①穴方一头针平刺快速进针,用小幅度快频率捻转,行针2分钟,每10分钟行针1次;②穴方二采用丝竹空穴透率谷法。得气后选取主穴中的2～4个穴位,接电针仪,使用疏密波,频率为2～100Hz,刺激强度以病人耐受为度,余穴每隔10分钟行针1次。肾虚、气血不足型每次取2～4穴,施温针灸,每穴3壮	是( )否( )	否定理由: 1. 频率: 2. 手法: 3. 其他原因及建议:
疗程:每次留针30分钟,头针可留至1小时。治疗频率隔日1次,10次为1疗程	是( )否( )	否定理由:

是否推荐针灸综合疗法
1. 强推荐( )2. 弱推荐( )3. 强不推荐( )4. 弱不推荐( )
如果选择3. 强不推荐或4. 弱不推荐,请您说明理由:

第三部分:方案排序
虽然各组方案中评价结局指标不尽相同,请您根据临床经验并针对临床证据,对上述疗法进行推荐排序:
急性期:A. 针刺(电针)治疗;B. 放血治疗;C. 火针治疗
对本《指南》推荐方案的其他批评意见:
专家信息表

专家姓名(电子签名)		年龄	
学历		专业	
职务		职称	
工作单位		工作年限	

您对针灸治疗偏头痛的熟悉程度是以下哪种情况？请在相应选项后标"√"

很熟悉	熟悉	一般	不熟悉	很不熟悉

您临床中使用针灸治疗偏头痛一般依据以下哪些？请在相应选项后标"√"，可以多选

A 教科书	B 现代文献	C 古代文献	D 名老中医经验	E 个人经验	F 师徒传承经验

G 其他 _____（请写明）

感谢您的指导与参与！

8 专家意见征集过程、结果汇总及处理

本《指南》在研制过程中，根据《针灸临床实践指南制定及评估规范》的要求，在循证基础上，充分吸取专家意见并尊重其指导作用，结合本《指南》研制过程中各个阶段、相应内容及遇到的争议问题，因需采取专家座谈、组内会议，并利用邮件、电话等较为灵活的不同方式，开展专家意见征集。详情如下：

8.1 《指南》适用范围的确定

《指南》的适用范围是指《指南》适用的疾病、状况及目标人群。本《指南》经过前期临床文献、名老中医著作调研，以及相关在研课题的考察，并通过召开组内专家会的形式，确定《指南》适用疾病为偏头痛，由于先兆偏头痛和无先兆偏头痛在偏头痛中占绝大多数，且在相关针治文献中，绝大部分针对这两型，故《指南》仅针对这两型偏头痛进行针灸治疗方案推荐。其他类型偏头痛，或其他原发和继发性头痛，也可参考推荐方案辨证施治。

8.2 《指南》临床问题的确定

在编写组整理提出临床问题基础上，通过召开组内专家会的形式，由专家组提炼确定。（具体内容见编写说明2. 临床问题）

8.3 证据的收集与评估

文献检索策略的制定：通过专家座谈、电子邮件等方式，确定了现代文献、古代文献的检索词、检索策略及检索数据库等。

文献质量评估：现代文献主要采用GRADE软件进行质量评价，由2位评估员分别评价，如有异议，提请专家组审核，通过组内专家会议定夺。

8.4 证据的合成及推荐方案的形成

由《指南》组长和专家组成员根据《指南》的适用范围和临床问题确定了本《指南》的编写框架。根据偏头痛的特点，将偏头痛分为发作期和缓解期，兼顾轻重程度、中医辨证分型。根据不同的分期写明适用的针灸疗法。本《指南》涉及的针灸疗法有：放血、针刺（电针）、火针、艾灸等。

8.5 形成推荐方案初稿及专家共识

由编写组召开专家会议，逐条对针灸治疗疾病的介入时机、适用人群、治疗原则、各种针灸方法及其疗效及安全性等进行讨论，筛选推荐方案，产生推荐意见。专家组在产生推荐意见时，充分考虑治疗方案的疗效、安全性和实用性。每一条推荐方案逐条根据以上原则产生。

8.6 修订推荐方案

确定征询意见专家范围：由编写小组结合专家组意见，在全国范围内遴选具有经验的针灸临床专家，职称为副主任医师或副教授以上，数量62名。

专家咨询的形式和内容：编写组将推荐方案通过电子邮件、纸质文本发放回收的形式，向咨询专家进行意见征集，请专家根据临床具体情况，对各推荐方案的原则、取穴、操作、疗程等各方面进行筛选和排序，并分别注明筛选和排序的原因。

8.7 修订和完善推荐方案

在2008年版偏头痛指南的基础上，对更新文献进行检索，用GRADE系统对全部纳入文献进行重新评价及证据等级的确定，在此基础上形成了新的证据，并就推荐方案进行修订。通过《指南》专家组成员的会议讨论，对推荐方案进行修订和完善。

9 会议纪要

9.1 2013年针灸临床实践指南项目审查会会议纪要

时间：2013年9月28日。

地点：成都。

参会人员：国家中医药管理局、中国针灸学会的有关领导，以及全国针灸行业的科、教、研各方

面共 26 名专家出席了会议，此外，还有 20 余名标准及指南起草单位的代表参加了会议。会议由中国针灸学会会长，全国针灸标准化技术委员会、中国针灸学会标准化工作委员会（以下简称"两针标委会"）主任委员刘保延主持，刘炜宏副主任委员、余曙光副主任委员分别担任 28 日上午和下午两个时间段的审查专家组组长。

会议内容：

国家中医药管理局政策法规与监督司查德忠司长到会并做了重要讲话。查司长在讲话中指出，标准化工作是国家中医药管理局法监司的工作重点，受到各方面的重视，局里已陆续出台一系列关于标准化工作的意义、规划及管理办法的文件以指导相关工作，同时已得到中央财政设中医标准化专款支持标准化项目。查司长鼓励针灸行业继续积极开展标准化工作，争取长久进展，他特别强调，要重视针灸标准体系和针灸标准化支撑体系的构建，要将针灸标准的制定与应用相结合，将标准的评价与应用相结合，要积极推进针灸标准化培训工作。在讲话最后，查司长提出了四点建议：一是要继续完善针灸标准化体系框架；二是要加强标准通则的制定；三是要围绕针灸临床实践来制定标准；四是要夯实针灸标准制定的基础。

中国针灸学会会长刘保延代表学会及两针标委会介绍了参加本次审查会的 2 项针灸国家标准、1 项针灸学会标准以及 15 项针灸临床实践指南项目的实施情况。在两针标委会的组织下，该 18 项标准（指南）的编制过程，严格遵循国家标准化管理委员会及中国针灸学会有关规定。目前，各项目组已对标准（指南）草案在全国范围内广泛征求意见，在今年 6 月份召开的两针标委会 2013 年年会上，该 18 项标准（指南）草案已通过初审。本次会议受国家中医药管理局委托，由两针标委会组织专家对标准（指南）送审稿进行审查。刘保延会长特别强调，临床实践指南是未来针灸标准化工作的重点，其性质更加贴近临床，其研制目的是为临床疗效和质量提供保障，所以，本次审订会上，针灸临床实践指南的评审重点是推荐方案的实用性。刘保延会长特请本次审查委员会专家严格把关，以确保标准（指南）的质量，他希望没有通过审查的项目起草单位能够做好修改和完善工作。

本次审查会对提交大会的 2 项针灸国家标准、1 项学会标准及 15 项针灸临床实践指南进行了审议，根据专家评审意见及专家投票情况得出评审结果：通过国家标准 1 项、学会标准 1 项、行业指南 6 项；建议修改后函审的行业指南 3 项；建议修改后会审的国家标准 1 项；未通过的行业指南 6 项。具体情况如下：

（1）审议通过的项目

专家审查委员会审查通过了由全国针灸标准化技术委员会起草的针灸国家标准《针灸临床治疗指南制定及评估规范》，由湖北中医药大学起草的中国针灸学会标准《针刀基本技术操作规范》，由中国中医科学院广安门医院起草的《慢性便秘针灸临床实践指南》和《腰痛针灸临床实践指南》，由北京中医药大学东直门医院起草的《原发性痛经针灸临床实践指南》，由成都中医药大学起草的《坐骨神经痛针灸临床实践指南》，由中国中医科学院针灸研究所起草的《失眠针灸临床实践指南》和《支气管哮喘（成人）针灸临床实践指南》。

（2）修改后函审的项目

由中国中医科学院针灸研究所起草的《肩周炎针灸临床实践指南》、由天津中医药大学起草的《膝骨性关节炎针灸临床实践指南》以及由北京中医药大学东直门医院起草的《过敏性鼻炎针灸临床实践指南》3 项指南，建议按照评审意见修订后再行函审。

（3）修改后会审的项目

由南京中医药大学起草的针灸国家标准《针灸门诊服务规范》，建议按照评审意见修订后再行会审。

（4）未通过的项目

由安徽中医学院附属针灸医院起草的《神经根型颈椎病针灸临床实践指南》、由天津中医药大学起草的《慢性萎缩性胃炎针灸临床实践指南》、由南京中医药大学起草的《突发性耳聋针灸临床实践指南》和《单纯性肥胖病针灸临床实践指南》、由浙江中医药大学附属医院起草的《原发性三叉神经痛针灸临床实践指南》以及由陕西中医学院起草的《糖尿病周围神经病变针灸临床实践指南》6项指南课题未通过审查。未通过审查的课题组按照评审意见继续修改和完善指南草案，由两针标委会秘书处另行安排验收审查。

最后，专家审查委员会提出，对于审议通过的标准，还需要对其内容及形式进行一致性修改，各标准起草单位应按照本次会议审查意见进行修改后，形成标准报批稿，上报两针标委会秘书处，经收集、整理、审核后，上报有关部门批准、发布。

9.2 2014年针灸临床实践指南项目审查会会议纪要

2014年3月6日，全国针灸标准化技术委员会、中国针灸学会标准化工作委员会在北京中国中医科学院广安门中医院组织召开了"2014年针灸标准及临床实践指南项目审查会"，会上审查了《偏头痛针灸临床实践指南再修订》（送审稿）。专家组经过认真评议形成如下意见：

本标准针对偏头痛针灸临床实践，通过收集整理偏头痛针灸临床实践和科研的相关文献资料、调研分析、专家论证，以古今文献、临床实践为依据，详细规定了该《指南》简介、疾病概述、临床特点、诊断标准、治疗概况、针灸治疗、推荐方案、附件等方面，形成了《偏头痛针灸临床实践指南》，并广泛征求专家意见、合理处理分析相关意见，达成了共识。

专家组一致认为本针灸临床实践指南编写方法符合标准化的有关规定，资料完整，用语确切，格式规范；《指南》框架及内容系统实用，具有科学性和可行性；偏头痛针灸临床治疗推荐方案合理，具备公认性和适用性；规定的针灸临床实践指南要求符合当前的科技水平和发展方向。

专家提出如下修订建议：

1. 疗效评价指标的分级还需要结合临床实际再细化。

2. 有几篇高质量英文文献的 GRADE 评级过低，需再重新评定。

3. 临床治疗方案还需根据临床可操作性进一步细化。

4. 审查组同意该《指南》通过审查。建议根据专家意见修改后，以行业标准上报审批。

附：《偏头痛针灸临床实践指南》项目评审专家名单

序号	姓名	职称/职务	工作单位
1	刘保延	副院长	中国中医科学院
2	刘炜宏	编审	中国中医科学院针灸所
3	文碧玲	教授	中国针灸学会
4	武晓冬	副研究员	中国中医科学院针灸所
5	余曙光	副校长/研究员	成都中医药大学
6	郭 义	教授	天津中医药大学
7	杨 骏	院长/教授	安徽中医学院
8	赵京生	研究员	中国中医科学院针灸所
9	杨华元	教授	上海中医药大学
10	储浩然	主任医师	安徽省针灸医院
11	石 现	主任医师	解放军总医院针灸科
12	王富春	院长/教授	长春中医药大学针灸推拿学院

序号	姓名	职称/职务	工作单位
13	王麟鹏	主任医师	首都医科大学附属北京市中医院
14	贾春生	主任医师	河北医科大学中医学院
15	余晓阳	主任医师	重庆市中医院
16	高希言	教授	河南中医学院
17	常小荣	教授	湖南中医药大学
18	张洪涛	主任医师	甘肃省中医院
19	吕明庄	主任医师	贵州省贵阳医学院附属医院
20	王玲玲	院长/教授	南京中医药大学
21	宣丽华	主任医师	浙江中医药大学附属第一医院
22	翟伟	教授	内蒙古医科大学中医学院